PET in the Aging Brain

Guest Editors

ANDREW B. NEWBERG, MD
ABASS ALAVI, MD,
MD (Hon), PhD (Hon), DSc (Hon)

PET CLINICS

www.pet.theclinics.com

Consulting Editor
ABASS ALAVI, MD,
MD (Hon), PhD (Hon), DSc (Hon)

January 2010 • Volume 5 • Number 1

SAUNDERS an imprint of ELSEVIER, Inc.

W.B. SAUNDERS COMPANY
A Division of Elsevier Inc.

1600 John F. Kennedy Boulevard • Suite 1800 • Philadelphia, Pennsylvania 19103-2899

http://www.theclinics.com

PET CLINICS Volume 5, Number 1
January 2010 ISSN 1556-8598, ISBN-13: 978-1-4377-1941-3

Editor: Barton Dudlick

PET Clinics (ISSN 1556-8598) is published quarterly by Elsevier Inc., 360 Park Avenue South, New York, NY 10010-1710. Months of issue are January, April, July, and October. Periodicals postage paid at New York, NY, and additional mailing offices. Subscription prices per year are $196.00 (US individuals), $279.00 (US institutions), $97.00 (US students), $223.00 (Canadian individuals), $312.00 (Canadian institutions), $118.00 (Canadian students), $237.00 (foreign individuals), $312.00 (foreign institutions), and $118.00 (foreign students). To receive student and resident rate, orders must be accompanied by name of affiliated institution, date of term, and the signature of program/residency coordinator on institution letterhead. Orders will be billed at individual rate until proof of status is received. Foreign air speed delivery is included in all Clinics subscription prices. All prices are subject to change without notice. POSTMASTER: Send address changes to PET Clinics, Elsevier Health Sciences Division, Subscription Customer Service, 3251 Riverport Lane, Maryland Heights, MO 63043. **Customer Service: 1-800-654-2452 (U.S. and Canada); 314-447-8871 (outside U.S. and Canada). Fax: 314-447-8029. E-mail: journalscustomerservice-usa@elsevier.com (for print support); journalsonlinesupport-usa@elsevier.com (for online support).**

Reprints. For copies of 100 or more of articles in this publication, please contact the Commercial Reprints Department, Elsevier Inc., 360 Park Avenue South, New York, NY 10010-1710. Tel.: 212-633-3812; Fax: 212-462-1935; E-mail: reprints@elsevier.com.

Printed and bound in the United Kingdom
Transferred to Digital Print 2011

Contributors

CONSULTING EDITOR

ABASS ALAVI, MD, MD (Hon), PhD (Hon), DSc (Hon)
Director of Research Education, Nuclear Medicine Section, Department of Radiology, Hospital of the University of Pennsylvania, Philadelphia, Pennsylvania

GUEST EDITORS

ANDREW B. NEWBERG, MD
Associate Professor, Division of Nuclear Medicine, Department of Radiology, University of Pennsylvania School of Medicine, Philadelphia, Pennsylvania

ABASS ALAVI, MD, MD (Hon), PhD (Hon), DSc (Hon)
Director of Research Education, Nuclear Medicine Section, Department of Radiology, Hospital of the University of Pennsylvania, Philadelphia, Pennsylvania

AUTHORS

ABASS ALAVI, MD, MD (Hon), PhD (Hon), DSc (Hon)
Director of Research Education, Nuclear Medicine Section, Department of Radiology, Hospital of the University of Pennsylvania, Philadelphia, Pennsylvania

V. BERTI, MD
Department of Psychiatry, Center for Brain Health, Silberstein Alzheimer's Institute, Center of Excellence on Brain Aging, NYU Langone Medical Center, New York, New York; Department of Clinical Pathophysiology, Nuclear Medicine Unit, University of Florence, Florence, Italy

ALAN P. CARPENTER, PhD, JD
Avid Radiopharmaceuticals Inc, Philadelphia, Pennsylvania

CHRISTOPHER M. CLARK, MD
Avid Radiopharmaceuticals Inc; Departments of Neurology and Radiology, University of Pennsylvania, Philadelphia, Pennsylvania

M.J. DE LEON, EdD
Department of Psychiatry, Center for Brain Health, Silberstein Alzheimer's Institute, Center of Excellence on Brain Aging, NYU Langone Medical Center, New York, New York; Nathan Kline Institute, Orangeburg, New York

S. DE SANTI, PhD
Department of Psychiatry, Center for Brain Health, Silberstein Alzheimer's Institute, Center of Excellence on Brain Aging, NYU Langone Medical Center, New York, New York

DAVID EIDELBERG, MD
Departments of Neurology and Medicine, North Shore University Hospital, Manhasset, New York

L. GLODZIK, MD, PhD
Department of Psychiatry, Center for Brain Health, Silberstein Alzheimer's Institute, Center of Excellence on Brain Aging, NYU Langone Medical Center, New York, New York

FRANZ F. HEFTI, PhD
Avid Radiopharmaceuticals Inc, Philadelphia, Pennsylvania

MICHAEL R. KILBOURN, PhD
Professor, Department of Radiology, University of Michigan, Ann Arbor, Michigan

HANK F. KUNG, PhD
Professor, Department of Radiology, University of Pennsylvania, Philadelphia, Pennsylvania

Y. LI, MD
Department of Psychiatry, Center for Brain Health, Silberstein Alzheimer's Institute, Center of Excellence on Brain Aging, NYU Langone Medical Center, New York, New York

L. MOSCONI, PhD
Department of Psychiatry, Center for Brain Health, Silberstein Alzheimer's Institute, Center of Excellence on Brain Aging, NYU Langone Medical Center, New York, New York

JAMES M. MOUNTZ, MD, PhD
Professor of Radiology; Chief of Nuclear Medicine and Director NeuroNuclear Medicine, University of Pittsburgh Medical Center, PET Facility, Pittsburgh, Pennsylvania

ANDREW B. NEWBERG, MD
Associate Professor, Division of Nuclear Medicine, Department of Radiology, University of Pennsylvania School of Medicine, Philadelphia, Pennsylvania

R.S. OSORIO, MD
Department of Psychiatry, Center for Brain Health; Departments of Pathology and Psychiatry, Alzheimer's Disease Center, Silberstein Alzheimer's Institute, Center of Excellence on Brain Aging, NYU Langone Medical Center, New York, New York; Alzheimer's Disease Research Unit, CIEN Foundation-Reina Sofia Foundation, Carlos III Institute of Health, Madrid, Spain

KATHLEEN L. POSTON, MD, MS
Department of Neurology and Neurological Sciences, Stanford University Medical Center, Stanford, California

WILLIAM J. POWERS, MD
H. Houston Merritt Distinguished Professor and Chair, Department of Neurology, University of North Carolina School of Medicine, Chapel Hill, North California

CHRISTOPHER C. ROWE, MD
Director, Department of Nuclear Medicine and Centre for PET, Austin Health; Professor, Department of Medicine, Austin Health, Victoria, Australia

JOHN P. SEIBYL, MD
Senior Scientist, Institute for Neurodegenerative Disorders, Molecular Neuroimaging, LLC, Yale University School of Medicine, New Haven, Connecticut

DANIEL M. SKOVRONSKY, MD, PhD
Avid Radiopharmaceuticals Inc; Department of Radiology, University of Pennsylvania, Philadelphia, Pennsylvania

VICTOR L. VILLEMAGNE, MD
Senior Research Fellow, Department of Nuclear Medicine and Centre for PET, Austin Health; Honorary Senior Research Officer, The Mental Health Research Institute of Victoria; Senior Research Fellow, Department of Medicine, Austin Health, Victoria, Australia

ALLYSON R. ZAZULIA, MD
Associate Professor, Departments of Neurology and Radiology, Washington University School of Medicine, St Louis, Missouri

Contents

Andrew B. Newberg and Abass Alavi

One of the most important aspects for the evaluation of PET brain scans for research or clinical purposes is to be able to identify normal variants. This article reviews issues pertaining to the technical and neurophysiologic aspects of functional brain imaging that might alter "normal" activity as evaluated by PET imaging. This includes an evaluation of various types of radiopharmaceuticals that measure cerebral blood flow, cerebral metabolism, and neurotransmitter activity. The baseline state of the brain and normal activity patterns associated with cognitive, sensory, and emotional processes are discussed in this article. In addition, the changes in the brain that occur during the life span of normal individuals are also considered because there is a different "normal" for each stage of life.

R.S. Osorio, V. Berti, L. Mosconi, Y. Li, L. Glodzik, S. De Santi, and M.J. de Leon

Early diagnosis of Alzheimer disease (AD) is one of the major challenges for the prevention of this dementia. The pathologic lesions associated with AD develop many years before the clinical manifestations of the disease become evident, during a likely transitional period between normal aging and the appearance of first cognitive symptoms. AD biomarkers are needed not only to reveal these early pathologic changes but also to monitor progression in cognitive and behavioral decline and brain lesions. PET neuroimaging can reliably assess indirect and direct aspects of the molecular biology and neuropathology of AD. This article reviews the use of [18F] 2-fluoro-2-deoxy-D-glucose–PET and amyloid PET imaging in the early detection of AD.

Victor L. Villemagne and Christopher C. Rowe

The progressive nature of neurodegeneration suggests an age-dependent process that ultimately leads to synaptic failure and neuronal damage in cortical areas of the brain critical for memory and higher mental functions. The increasing age of the population in developed countries suggests that, if unchecked, these disorders will become increasingly prevalent. In the absence of specific biologic markers, direct pathologic examination of brain tissue still is the only definitive method for establishing a diagnosis of Alzheimer disease (AD) and other types of dementia. Pathologic hallmarks of AD are intracellular neurofibrillary tangles (NFT) and extracellular amyloid plaques. NFT are intraneuronal bundles of paired helical filaments mainly composed of the aggregates of an abnormally phosphorylated form of tau protein; neuritic plaques consist of dense extracellular aggregates of β-amyloid (Aβ), surrounded by reactive gliosis and dystrophic neurites. To date, all available evidence strongly supports the notion that an imbalance between the production and removal of Aβ leading to its progressive accumulation is central to the pathogenesis of AD. A growing understanding of the molecular mechanisms of Aβ formation, degradation, and neurotoxicity is being translated into new therapeutic approaches. Whereas AD is the most common cause of dementia in the elderly, postmortem studies have found dementia with Lewy Bodies and frontotemporal lobe degeneration each to account for about 20% of cases. Molecular neuroimaging techniques such as PET have been used for the in vivo assessment of molecular processes at their sites of action, permitting detection of subtle pathophysiological changes in the brain at asymptomatic stages The development of molecular imaging methods for noninvasively assessing disease-specific traits such as Aβ burden in AD is allowing early diagnosis at presymptomatic stages, more accurate differential diagnosis and, when available, the evaluation and monitoring of disease-modifying therapy.

Network analysis of ^{18}F-fluorodeoxyglucose (FDG) PET is an innovative approach for the study of movement disorders such as Parkinson disease (PD). Spatial covariance analysis of imaging data acquired from PD patients has revealed characteristic regional patterns associated with the motor and cognitive features of disease. Quantification of pattern expression in individual patients can be used for diagnosis, assessment of disease severity, and evaluation of novel medical and surgical therapies. Identification of disease-specific patterns in other parkinsonian syndromes, such as multiple system atrophy and progressive supranuclear palsy, has improved diagnostic accuracy in patients with parkinsonism that is difficult to diagnose. Further developments of these techniques are likely to enhance the role of functional imaging in investigating underlying abnormalities and potential new therapies in these neurodegenerative diseases.

Parkinson disease (PD) is the prototypic movement disorder originally described by James Parkinson, and it accounts for about 80% of a group of related degenerative motor disorders collectively referred to as the parkinsonisms, Parkinson spectrum disorders, or Parkinson plus disorders, terms which are used interchangeably throughout this article. Much work with positron emission tomography (PET) and single-photon emission computed tomography (SPECT) in the movement disorders has focused on the dopamine system. There have been at least 3 different presynaptic dopaminergic targets that are used successfully to interrogate this system. Another approach may be is to assess the dynamics of dopamine release into the synapse by the use of reversible-bound PET tracers or SPECT tracers. Both dopaminergic and nondopaminergic imaging in the diagnosis of movement disorders are discussed in this article.

The early detection and monitoring of neurodegenerative diseases, including Parkinson disease, Alzheimer disease, dementia with Lewy bodies and other dementias, and movement disorders, represent a significant unmet medical need. Tools for accurate and early differential diagnosis are necessary to determine the appropriate treatment for patients and to minimize inappropriate use of potentially harmful treatments. Such diagnostic imaging tools are expected to permit monitoring of disease progression and will thus accelerate testing and development of disease-modifying drugs. The new imaging tests may be useful as prognostic tools by identifying humans with neurodegenerative diseases before the clinical manifestations become evident.

Investigation of the interplay between the cerebral circulation and brain cellular function is fundamental to understanding both the pathophysiology and treatment of stroke. At present, PET is the only technique that provides accurate, quantitative in vivo regional measurements of both cerebral circulation and cellular metabolism in human subjects. This article reviews normal human cerebral blood flow and metabolism, and human PET studies of ischemic stroke, carotid artery disease, vascular dementia, intracerebral hemorrhage, and aneurysmal subarachnoid hemorrhage, and discusses how these studies have added to the understanding of the pathophysiology of human cerebrovascular disease.

Use of imaging with the objective of improvement of stroke recovery should have a significant impact on determination of prognosis for recovery, which should assist patients and families in coping with the disabilities secondary to a stroke and assist in long-term planning for the disposition and needs of the patient. Serial evaluation of stroke physiology and presence or absence of cerebral reorganization by imaging techniques provide a rationale for development of physical rehabilitation strategies based on implementation of adaptive plasticity models and allow patient selection into more individualized rehabilitation treatment programs, emphasizing facilitatory versus compensatory techniques.

PET Clinics

THE CLINICS ARE NOW AVAILABLE ONLINE!

Access your subscription at:
www.theclinics.com

GOAL STATEMENT

The goal of the *PET Clinics* is to keep practicing radiologists and radiology residents up to date with current clinical practice in positron emission tomography by providing timely articles reviewing the state of the art in patient care.

ACCREDITATION

PET Clinics is planned and implemented in accordance with the Essential Areas and Policies of the Accreditation Council for Continuing Medical Education (ACCME) through the joint sponsorship of the University of Virginia School of Medicine and Elsevier. The University of Virginia School of Medicine is accredited by the ACCME to provide continuing medical education for physicians.

The University of Virginia School of Medicine designates this educational activity for a maximum of 15 *AMA PRA Category 1 Credits*™ for each issue, 60 credits per year. Physicians should only claim credit commensurate with the extent of their participation in the activity.

The American Medical Association has determined that physicians not licensed in the US who participate in this CME activity are eligible for a maximum of 15 *AMA PRA Category 1 Credits*™ for each issue, 60 credits per year.

Category 1 credit can be earned by reading the text material, taking the CME examination online at http://www.theclinics.com/home/cme, and completing the evaluation. After taking the test, you will be required to review any and all incorrect answers. Following completion of the test and evaluation, your credit will be awarded and you may print your certificate.

FACULTY DISCLOSURE/CONFLICT OF INTEREST

The University of Virginia School of Medicine, as an ACCME accredited provider, endorses and strives to comply with the Accreditation Council for Continuing Medical Education (ACCME) Standards of Commercial Support, Commonwealth of Virginia statutes, University of Virginia policies and procedures, and associated federal and private regulations and guidelines on the need for disclosure and monitoring of proprietary and financial interests that may affect the scientific integrity and balance of content delivered in continuing medical education activities under our auspices.

The University of Virginia School of Medicine requires that all CME activities accredited through this institution be developed independently and be scientifically rigorous, balanced and objective in the presentation/discussion of its content, theories and practices.

All authors/editors participating in an accredited CME activity are expected to disclose to the readers relevant financial relationships with commercial entities occurring within the past 12 months (such as grants or research support, employee, consultant, stock holder, member of speakers bureau, etc.). The University of Virginia School of Medicine will employ appropriate mechanisms to resolve potential conflicts of interest to maintain the standards of fair and balanced education to the reader. Questions about specific strategies can be directed to the Office of Continuing Medical Education, University of Virginia School of Medicine, Charlottesville, Virginia.

The faculty and staff of the University of Virginia Office of Continuing Medical Education have no financial affiliations to disclose.

The authors/editors listed below have identified no professional or financial affiliations for themselves or their spouse/partner:
Abass Alavi, MD, MD(Hon), PhD(Hon), DSc(Hon) (Consulting and Guest Editor); V. Berti, MD; Barton Dudlick (Acquisitions Editor); David Eidelberg, MD; Y. Li, MD; L. Mosconi, PhD; James M. Mountz, MD, PhD; Andrew B. Newberg, MD (Guest Editor); R.S. Osorio, MD; Kathleen L. Poston, MD, MS; Patrice Rehm, MD (Test Author); and Allyson R. Zazulia, MD.

The authors/editors listed below identified the following professional or financial affiliations for themselves or their spouse/partner:
Alan P. Carpenter, PhD, JD is employed by and owns stock in Avid Radiopharmaceuticals.
Christopher Clark, MD is employed by and owns stock in Avid Radiopharmaceuticals.
M.J. de Leon, EdD holds a patent with Abient technologies.
S. De Santi, PhD is an industry funded research/investigator and is on the Advisory Committee/Board for Bayer Healthcare Pharmaceuticals, and is a consultant for The Cognition Group.
L. Glodzik, MD, PhD is an industry funded research/investigator for Forest Lab.
Franz F. Hefti, PhD is employed by and owns stock in Avid Radiopharmaceuticals.
Michael R. Kilbourn, PhD is on the Advisory Committee/Board for Avid Radiopharmaceuticals.
Hank F. Kung, PhD is an industry funded research/investigator and consultant, and is on the Speakers' Bureau for Avid Radiopharmaceuticals, Inc.
William J. Powers, MD is a consultant for Certus International.
Christopher C. Rowe, MD is a consultant for Bayer Schering Pharma.
John P. Seibyl, MD is a consultant for GE Healthcare, is an industry funded research/investigator for Bayer Healthcare and Eli Lilly, and owns stock in Molecular Neuroimaging.
Daniel M. Skovronsky, MD, PhD is employed by, is on the Advisory Committee/Board of, owns stock in, and holds a patent for, Avid Radiopharmaceuticals.
Victor L. Villemagne, MD is a consultant for Bayer Schering Pharma.

Disclosure of Discussion of Non-FDA Approved Uses for Pharmaceutical Products and/or Medical Devices.
The University of Virginia School of Medicine, as an ACCME provider, requires that all faculty presenters identify and disclose any off-label uses for pharmaceutical and medical device products. The University of Virginia School of Medicine recommends that each physician fully review all the available data on new products or procedures prior to clinical use.

TO ENROLL

To enroll in the PET Clinics Continuing Medical Education program, call customer service at 1-800-654-2452 or visit us online at www.theclinics.com/home/cme.**The CME program is available to subscribers for an additional fee of $196.00.**

Preface

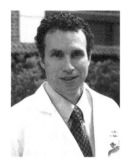
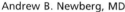
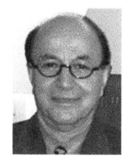

Andrew B. Newberg, MD   Abass Alavi, MD, MD (Hon),
                                      PhD (Hon), DSc (Hon)
Guest Editors

The use of PET has presented an important and unique opportunity for investigating neuropsychiatric disorders. PET imaging began with the development of ^{18}F-fluorodeoxyglucose (FDG) but has grown to include a multitude of radiopharmaceuticals that can evaluate almost any aspect of brain function. Emission tomography to image the biodistribution of radionuclides was originally developed in the 1960s by David Kuhl and Roy Edwards. This technique was later named single-photon emission computed tomography (SPECT) and was used to study several neurologic disorders as well as to accurately demonstrate the regional distribution of various tracers in the central nervous system. SPECT studies use single photon-emitting radionuclides, such as iodine or technetium, that are labeled to a specific compound. Concurrent with these developments, it was realized that positron-emitting radionuclides allow for the synthesis of biologically important radiotracers because the elements used for labeling are identical or close to those that are naturally contained in such compounds. Thus, radionuclides such as ^{11}C, ^{18}F, and ^{13}N seem useful in producing a vast array of tracers that are optimal for studying the brain's chemistry and function. The emitted positron travels a short distance before meeting an electron and annihilating to produce 2 511-keV γ-rays, which travel in opposite directions, approximately 180° from each other. Modern whole-body PET instruments

have a resolution in the range of 3 to 4 mm. This resolution has approached the theoretic limit of a few millimeters, resulting in considerable improvement of image quality. Thus, PET is primed to be able to contribute substantially to the understanding of neuropsychiatric conditions in the future.

Over the past 35 years, PET imaging has been used to evaluate regional cerebral glucose metabolism in clinical and research applications. The array of disorders that have been studied include neurologic disorders, such as dementia, stroke, brain tumors, movement disorders, and seizures, and psychiatric disorders, including schizophrenia, mood disorders, anxiety, and drug abuse. One major development, which revealed the ability of PET in elucidating regional brain metabolism and function, was the synthesis of FDG. The early work performed with FDG-PET had explored the metabolic landscape and changes associated with various neuropsychiatric disorders. This greatly advanced the understanding of these disorders and the particular brain structures affected. Recent work has focused more on clinical issues, including diagnosis, management, and follow-up. Studies have also attempted to ascertain predictors of response to therapeutic interventions and have explored how specific activation paradigms might help uncover specific deficits not apparent with resting images.

doi:10.1016/j.cpet.2010.03.002
1556-8598/10/$ – see front matter © 2010 Elsevier Inc. All rights reserved.

pet.theclinics.com

Over this same period of time, a wide array of radiopharmaceuticals has been developed. Tracers that can evaluate pre- and postsynaptic receptor function have been used to explore the dopamine, serotonin, glutamate, benzodiazepine, and opiate receptor systems. In addition, newer tracers have been developed that evaluate other pathophysiologic processes, such as amyloid deposition, hypoxia, and apoptosis. Each of these new tracers may have a variety of uses in the study of neuropsychiatric conditions.

The January and April issues of *PET Clinics* explore what PET imaging has revealed in a variety of neuropsychiatric disorders in research and clinical settings. The articles describe the current status of PET data in different disorders, reveal current progress in understanding these disorders, and provide a foundation for future studies. It is important to show this overall perspective so that PET imaging can continue to be a highly valuable tool in the study of brain and the disorders affecting the brain.

Andrew B. Newberg, MD

Abass Alavi, MD, MD (Hon), PhD (Hon), DSc (Hon)
Division of Nuclear Medicine
Department of Radiology
University of Pennsylvania School of Medicine
110 Donner Building
H.U.P., 3400 Spruce Street
Philadelphia, PA 19104, USA

E-mail addresses:
Andrew.newberg@uphs.upenn.edu (A.B. Newberg)
abass.alavi@uphs.upenn.edu (A. Alavi)

Normal Patterns and Variants in PET Brain Imaging

Andrew B. Newberg, MD*,
Abass Alavi, MD, MD (Hon), PhD (Hon), DSc (Hon)

KEYWORDS

- Radionuclide • Brain imaging • Neurotransmitter
- Metabolism • PET

One of the most important aspects for the evaluation of PET brain scans for research or clinical purposes is to be able to identify normal variants. For functional brain imaging in general, it is not always easy to characterize the term "normal" because many normal brain functions and mental activities might affect brain activity as measured by PET scans. This article reviews issues pertaining to the technical and neurophysiologic aspects of functional brain imaging that might alter "normal" activity as evaluated by PET imaging. This includes an evaluation of various types of radiopharmaceuticals that measure cerebral blood flow, cerebral metabolism, and neurotransmitter activity. The baseline state of the brain and normal activity patterns associated with cognitive, sensory, and emotional processes are discussed in this article. In addition, the changes in the brain that occur during the life span of normal individuals are also considered because there is a different "normal" for each stage of life.

Tomographic brain imaging was first developed in the 1960s by Kuhl and Edwards,[1] using single-photon emission computed tomography (SPECT), and was used to obtain the first transaxial reconstructions of radionuclide distribution in the brain. This technique was used to study several neurologic and psychiatric disorders and their effect on radionuclide distribution in the central nervous system (CNS).[2] SPECT was the first functional imaging modality that was used in the study of the CNS, and these early studies met with much success.[3] The SPECT studies used single-photon emitters, such as iodine 123 or technetium 99m, as radionuclides that would be attached to the substrate. Today, the most commonly used radioligands for SPECT to measure the blood flow are ^{99m}Tc hexamethyl propylene amine oxime and ^{99m}Tc ethyl cysteinate dimer. However, several radiopharmaceutical systems (**Tables 1** and **2**) for SPECT and PET imaging have been developed to study various aspects of cerebral function, including a wide array of neurotransmitters.[4,5] At the moment, none of the neurotransmitter studies are clinically available, but in the near future, neurotransmitter tracers are likely to play a larger role in the clinical evaluation of specific neuropsychiatric disorders.

Although SPECT was useful, it was realized that positron-emitting radionuclides would allow for more and better radiopharmaceuticals because the atoms used would be isotopes of elements that naturally occur in various organic molecules such as glucose, amino acids, or neurotransmitters. Thus, radionuclides such as ^{11}C, ^{18}F, and ^{13}N would be useful in producing a vast number of tracers that could be used for studying body chemistry and function.[3] Investigators from Brookhaven National Laboratory, in collaboration with those from the University of Pennsylvania, were the first to synthesize ^{18}F-fluorodeoxyglucose (FDG) that could be used for measuring regional cerebral glucose metabolism.[6] The emitted positron, from the decay of the ^{18}F atom, travels several millimeters before annihilating to produce two 511-keV gamma rays that travel in opposite

Division of Nuclear Medicine, Department of Radiology, University of Pennsylvania School of Medicine, 110 Donner Building, H.U.P., 3400 Spruce Street, Philadelphia, PA 19104, USA
* Corresponding author.
E-mail address: Andrew.Newberg@uphs.upenn.edu

PET Clin 5 (2010) 1–13
doi:10.1016/j.cpet.2009.12.006
1556-8598/10/$ – see front matter © 2010 Published by Elsevier Inc.

Table 1
A partial listing of radioligands used in neurologic SPECT imaging

Compound	Application
HMPAO, IMP, ECD	Cerebral blood flow
3-quinuclidinyl benzilate (IQNB)	Muscarinic cholinergic receptor
Iodopride, IBZM, iodospiperone	Dopamine receptor activity
AMIK, DOI	Serotonin receptor activity
Iomazenil	Benzodiazepine activity
2-iodomorphine	Opioid receptor activity
I-d(CH2)5[Tyr(Me)2, Tyr(NH2)9]AV	Vasopressin activity

AMIK, 7-amino-8-iodo-ketanserin; DOI, 1-(2,5-dimethoxy-4-iodiophenyl)-2-aminopropane; ECD, ethyl cysteinate dimer; HMPAO, 99mTc hexamethyl propylene amine oxime; IBZM, 3-iodo-N-[(1-ethyl-2-pyrrolidinyl)] menthyl-2-hydroxy-6-methoxybenzamide; IMP, Iodine-123-N-N', N, -trimethyl-N'-[2-hydroxyl-3-methyl-5-iodo-benzyl]-1, 3 propane diamine.

directions. Thus, PET has a theoretical limit of spatial resolution of 2 to 3 mm (compared with the resolution of SPECT, which is 8 to 10 mm) based on the positron's mean path length before annihilation. Significant progress has been made in the design and manufacture of PET instruments that are capable of generating transaxial image reconstruction close to the theoretical limit.[7–9]

The most commonly used radiopharmaceutical for neurologic PET imaging (see **Table 2**) is ^{18}F-FDG, which measures the cerebral metabolic rate for glucose (**Fig. 1**). FDG is currently the only approved tracer for the evaluation of brain function (specifically for seizure disorders), dementia, and brain tumors. FDG-PET has also been used to study a wide variety of neurologic disorders, such as dementia and psychiatric illness, and the effects of various stimulatory phenomena on the human CNS.[10,11] In addition to FDG, there has been the development of other positron-emitting

biochemical analogs for measuring a wide array of neurophysiologic processes. There have actually been only a limited number of studies that have attempted to discern normal variants and changes over time in the normal population.

NORMAL VARIANTS IN FUNCTIONAL NEUROIMAGING STUDIES

The ability to detect abnormalities on clinical brain scans or for research purposes initially requires a determination of the normal variations that might be observed on such scans. One of the primary issues related to the definition of "normal" that arises with brain imaging is the determination of the "baseline" brain state. There has been considerable attention in the literature regarding the best conditions to obtain a baseline functional imaging study. In particular, what the patient is doing and experiencing may have a profound influence on

Table 2
A partial listing of radioligands used in neurologic PET imaging

Compound	Application
[15O]H$_2$O	Blood flow
[18F]fluorodeoxyglucose	Glucose metabolism
[15O]O$_2$	Oxygen metabolism
[11C]L-methionine	Amino acid metabolism
[11C]raclopride, [11C]methylspiperone, 6-[18F]fluorodopamine, [18F]spiperone	Dopamine system
[11C](+)McN5652, [11C]DASB	Serotonin system
[11C]carfentanil, [11C]etorphine	Opiate system
[11C]flunitrazepam	Benzodiazepine system
[11C]scopolamine, [11C]quinuclidinyl benzilate	Muscarinic cholinergic receptors
[11C]ephedrine, [18F]fluorometaraminol	Adrenergic terminals
[11C]Pittsburgh Compound B, [18F]AV45, [18F]flutemetamol	Amyloid imaging

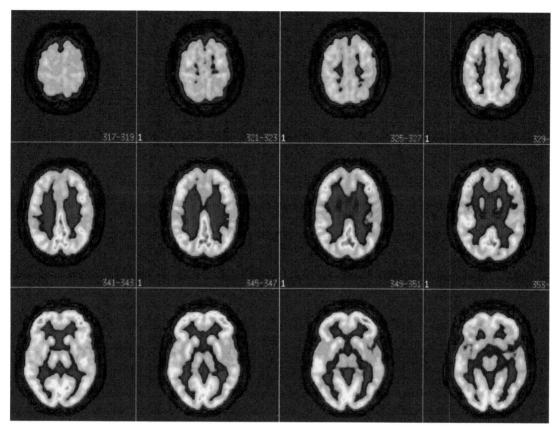

Fig. 1. Normal FDG-PET scan in a 45-year-old individual.

brain function. This has provided a foundation for activation studies that are typically performed on normal control subjects performing various sensorimotor, cognitive, or affective tasks. For example, the brain function with eyes open is markedly different compared with the brain function with eyes closed.[12] Once the eyes are open, there is a dramatic increase in the primary visual areas (**Fig. 2**). This activity increases with the complexity of the scene being presented to the brain.[13] Movement in the external environment also alters functions in the visual centers of the brain as well as in the medial prefrontal cortex, temporoparietal junction, basal temporal regions, and extrastriate cortex.[14,15] Sounds elicit changes in cerebral function and, whether the ears are occluded or not, may influence brain function. For example, PET studies have demonstrated that the processing of simple auditory stimuli, such as pure tones and noise, predominantly activates the left transverse temporal gyrus, whereas sounds with discontinued acoustic patterns, activated parts of the auditory association area in the superior temporal gyri, and complex sounds, such as words, speech, and music, activate extensive associative auditory areas in both hemispheres.[16,17]

Other areas of research related to normal variations in brain activity are cerebral activation studies of higher cognitive processes. During the past decade, many studies have explored the areas involved in attention; problem solving; and more recently, moral thinking and even religious practices, such as meditation.[18–20] Each of these tasks involves one or more areas of the brain and may result in areas of increased or decreased activity. For example, attention-focusing tasks

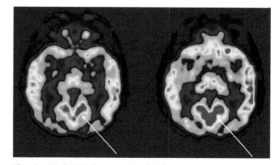

Fig. 2. FDG-PET in a normal subject with eyes closed (*left*) compared with that of the same individual with eyes open, revealing significantly greater occipital lobe activity (*arrow*), with the open eyes stimulating the primary visual cortex.

typically demonstrate increased activity in the prefrontal cortex and anterior cingulate gyrus.[21,22] Emotional responses frequently involve limbic structures, such as the amygdala, and various neurotransmitters.[23–25] Although these studies are extremely interesting for determining the neurophysiologic basis of such tasks and experiences, the results also have implications for routine clinical studies. The most directly relevant issue is what people should think about while being injected with the radiopharmaceutical. In an FDG-PET imaging of the whole body, typical findings of increased muscle activity are found in association with movement or tension in those muscle groups. If a person undergoing a brain scan is particularly anxious about a personal or health problem or is trying to solve a significant business problem, the results of the brain scan might be considerably different from those of a person undergoing a scan when he or she is more relaxed. Thus, the different cognitive and emotional states of a person at the time of a given study may result in "normal variants" of brain activity even though they actually signify particular mental processes.

Technical factors must also be considered when evaluating brain function because they may introduce artifacts and findings that are, in reality, variants of normal brain perfusion. These include the time between injection and scanning, the dose administered, filtering and processing steps, and test-retest variability. As the duration from the time of injection increases, it is possible that certain tracers may have an altered cerebral distribution, especially if they redistribute rapidly. The ideal tracer would remain completely fixed within the brain at the time of extraction. However, most tracers do experience some degree of washout and some even undergo substantial redistribution. Other tracers, especially neurotransmitters, may have altered biodistribution over time, and this is a factor that must be considered for any clinical or research study. PET tracers, with considerably shorter half-lives, must also be imaged relatively close to the time of injection. FDG images are typically obtained in 45 to 60 minutes. By virtue of decay, image quality and therefore sensitivity and specificity for detecting abnormalities likely decline if the imaging is significantly delayed. Short-lived isotopes, such as [^{15}O] H_2O, must be imaged at the time of the injection if any worthwhile images are to be obtained. Likewise, the dose administered potentially affects the quality of the study and the ability to evaluate more central structures.

Filtering and processing of the images is also crucial to determine cerebral activity. PET imaging requires appropriate filtering, attenuation correction, correction for random events, single photon detections, and dead time. Attenuation correction is necessary particularly for adequately visualizing and comparing activities in brain structures, especially deeper structures such as the thalamus or the brain stem (**Fig. 3**). Patient motion can always complicate interpretation of PET scans. Methods for preventing patient motion from interfering with scanning include firm head holders and the use of tape or some other method to hold the head in place. Also, the shortening of image acquisition time makes the session easier on the patient. Alternatively, breaking up of the acquisition time into multiple shorter scans can be useful because scans with motion can be excluded without losing the entire study. Current image acquisition and analysis software also provides postacquisition processing to correct the motion artifact. Another processing factor that can affect the visual inspection of brain scans is head tilt. Beacuse a patient's head is rarely in complete alignment with the scanner, significant head tilt might result in certain areas appearing asymmetric in comparison with the contralateral structure. For example, thalami can frequently seem to have asymmetric activity if there is head tilt. However, this can usually be identified by examining all of the slices containing the structure. As the slices proceed through the structure, asymmetries associated with head tilt should flip from one side to the other. This can usually be corrected by computer programs that realign brain images. However, being able to identify the tilt is an important initial step.

Despite many of these issues, most studies of cerebral blood flow, metabolism, or even neurotransmitter systems have demonstrated good test-retest reliability with small variability within structures.[26,27] Most studies have shown that in healthy controls, repeat scans typically demonstrate regional activity and absolute activity to be within 5% to 10%.

NEUROIMAGING IN THE STUDY OF NORMAL AGING FROM INFANCY TO ADULTHOOD

The normal aging process is associated with several biochemical changes in the brain. Although postmortem studies may help to elucidate the nature of these changes, the advent of functional neuroimaging techniques allows these biochemical changes in the brain to be measured in vivo across the life span of the person. PET imaging has been useful in the investigation of the normal development of pediatric subjects.[28,29] During the first year of normal development, studies have shown that the pattern of glucose

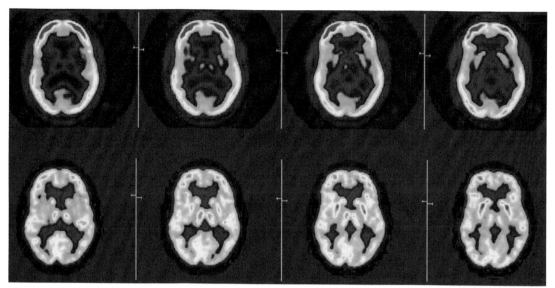

Fig. 3. Normal FDG-PET scans without (*top row*) and with (*bottom row*) attenuation correction. The noncorrected images show uniformly decreased metabolism throughout the central structures, which is markedly improved after attenuation correction.

metabolism generally corresponds to the phylogenetic order of development (**Fig. 4**). Thus, the functional maturation (as measured by increased metabolism) of developmentally older structures precedes that of structures that develop later.[30,31] Further, the pattern of glucose metabolism correlates with the manifestation of various behaviors in infants. For example, as the visuospatial and visuosensorimotor functions develop, increased glucose metabolism is observed in the parietal, temporal, cerebellar, and primary visual cortices. Increases have also been observed in the basal ganglia as movement and sensorimotor function become more integrated. Glucose metabolism in the frontal lobe remains low during the first 4 months of life and increases as the infant begins to develop higher cortical and cognitive capabilities.[28] Thus, as the infant develops more complex social interactions and improves its abilities in various neuropsychological tests that specifically involve frontal lobe function, these changes are reflected by gradual increases in the frontal lobe metabolic activity. By one year of age, the overall pattern of glucose metabolism is qualitatively similar to that of a young adult.[28] However, frontal lobe activity increases later in development than the other cortical areas.[32]

Despite the qualitative similarity in glucose metabolism, infants typically have markedly decreased metabolic rates compared with adults. Neonatal metabolic rates are approximately 30% of adult rates. The metabolic values increase until the third year, when the metabolism actually

surpasses adult values. The glucose metabolic rate plateaus near the age of 4 years until approximately age 9 years. This elevated metabolic value may be as high as 1.3 times that of normal young adults.[33] After age 9, the metabolic rate declines to adult values by the end of the second decade.[30] It has been suggested that the increased metabolism is the result of increased brain development and reorganization. This may reflect the increased activity for the overgrowth and elimination phases of neuronal development such that appropriate neuronal connections become manifested. For example, the decline of glucose metabolism in the visual cortex corresponds to the time when neuronal plasticity decreases.[28] It is this time that corresponds to the mature development of the visual system.

The results of functional brain imaging studies in normal aging have generally noted a global decrease in cerebral blood flow and metabolism with age.[34,35] This typically affects the gray matter more than the white matter.[36] Furthermore, the decrease seems to be nonlinear with a sharper decrease before the age of approximately 36 years, followed by a slower decline.[37] Although several areas seem to be affected, the most commonly observed decrease is in the frontal lobes bilaterally (**Fig. 5**). Regional cerebral blood flow has been reported to decrease in the frontal lobes bilaterally with increasing age.[38] A PET study by Martin and colleagues[39] also described decreases in regional cerebral blood flow in the cingulate gyrus, parahippocampal gyrus, superior

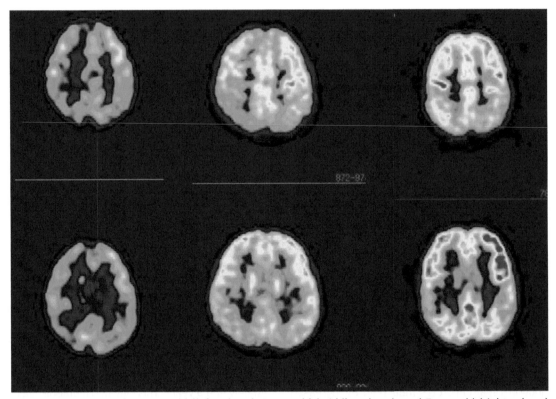

Fig. 4. FDG-PET scans of a 1-year-old (*left column*), 3-year-old (*middle column*), and 7-year-old (*right column*), revealing changing pattern of metabolism in the cortex. The 1-year-old has little metabolism in the cortex, whereas the 3-year-old and 7-year-old have progressively increased metabolism.

temporal lobe, medial frontal lobe, and posterior parietal cortex with increasing age. Overall, the areas with decreasing perfusion with age are the limbic system and the association areas. These authors suggested that these decreases might reflect the cognitive changes that occur with age. One study indicated that there was a significant age-related decrease in the cerebral blood flow in the left superior temporal area.[40] Although there does seem to be an overall decrease in cerebral blood flow with aging, there may be a predilection for the left hemisphere.[41] FDG-PET findings in normal aging in adults have generally reported a decrease in whole-brain cerebral metabolic rate for glucose (CMRGlc) values. Several investigators have described diminished regional glucose metabolism in the temporal, parietal, somatosensory, and especially the frontal regions.[42–46] A summary of regional metabolic changes observed in normal aging is shown in **Box 1**. Kuhl and colleagues[47] showed that there was a decrease in the mean CMRGlc with age. At age 78, there was a mean decrease of 26% in the CMRGlc compared with subjects at age 18. Alavi and colleagues[48] showed that there was a general decline in metabolic activities in the

frontal and somatosensory areas. Minor health problems seemed to have no significant effects on regional or whole-brain CMRGlc.

A more recent study[49] using high-resolution FDG-PET imaging in 120 healthy volunteers with ages ranging from 19 to 79 years found that the most consistent finding associated with normal aging was decreased cortical metabolism. The frontal lobe, in particular, showed decreased metabolism with age. Other cortical areas such as the parietal, occipital, and temporal areas showed marked variation within and across age groups. However, one study with a limited number of subjects suggested that the temporal lobe may also be particularly affected by the aging process.[50] These changes in metabolism are also reflected in an increased cerebellum-to-cortex ratio and an increased anterior-posterior metabolic gradient seen with advancing age.

Another finding based on functional neuroimaging studies is that the metabolic activities in the frontal, parietal, and occipital lobes seem to be symmetric regardless of age.[49] However, the left temporal lobe tends to be hypometabolic compared with the right temporal lobe. This remains true regardless of age. Cerebral

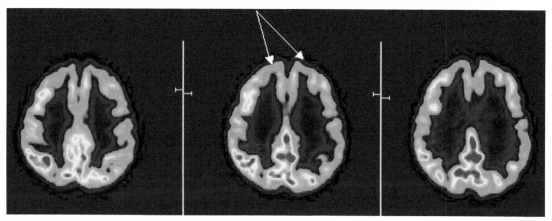

Fig. 5. FDG-PET scan of a patient with normal aging, revealing decreased metabolism throughout the frontal lobes (*arrows*).

metabolism in structures such as the basal ganglia, thalami, hippocampi, cerebellum, visual cortices, and posterior cingulate gyrus is relatively preserved throughout the later decades of life and remains symmetric.[49] The visual cortices generally tend to be hypermetabolic compared with the rest of the brain and remain so throughout the life span.[42,51] Earlier studies have shown that there were elevated ratios of visual cortex to whole brain in the elderly compared with controls, but later studies have not yet confirmed this.[49] Metabolic activity in the brain stem has been found to increase markedly with increasing age. Although the reason for this increase is unclear, it has been hypothesized that changes in neurotransmitter activity, such as in the dopaminergic system, may alter the metabolism in the brain stem.

Several studies have explored whether there are differences between men and women with regard to regional cerebral glucose metabolism and also how these values might change with age. An early PET study did not demonstrate any significant differences.[52] However, more recent studies have suggested that there are baseline differences between men and women and that the metabolic pattern changes with age differently, depending on the gender. For example, 1 PET study demonstrated that males had significantly higher glucose metabolism in the right insula, middle temporal gyrus, and medial frontal lobe than females.[53] However, glucose metabolism in the hypothalamus was significantly higher in females than in males. There was a significant correlation between aging and glucose metabolism in the left thalamus in males and in the left caudate nucleus and hypothalamus in females.

Given the initial studies showing a decrease in cerebral glucose metabolism with increasing age, it has been hypothesized that this finding might be related to the rate with which the radiopharmaceutical, FDG, is transported into the brain or is phosphorylated once inside the neurons. However, several reports[54,55] have showed that the decrease in cerebral metabolism was not related to these rate constants. Thus, the decrease in FDG uptake seems to correlate with an actual decrease in brain metabolism.

Dastur[56] reported no difference in the global cerebral metabolic rate of oxygen ($CMRO_2$) with normal aging. However, PET studies using the ^{15}O inhalation method have found decreases in $CMRO_2$ in the gray matter with increasing age.[57] Similarly, a significant decrease in the mean $CMRO_2$ has been observed in subjects older

---

Box 1
Regions observed to have significant hypometabolism with aging[a]

Frontal

    Anterior corpus callosum

    Cingulate gyrus

    Frontal pole

    Frontal eye fields

    Middle frontal gyrus

Temporal

    Middle temporal gyrus

Parietal

    Superior parietal gyrus

Sensorimotor

    Primary sensory cortex

[a] Regions of interest significant at $P = .001$.

than 51 years compared with subjects younger than 50 years.[40] Particular areas found to have decreased oxygen metabolism with age were the bilateral putamen, the left supratemporal, left infrafrontal, and left parietal cortices. As described earlier, decreases in cerebral blood flow have been observed in normal aging.[36,39] Other studies have not found a significant decrease in blood flow with aging[40] but have found that the decreases could not account for the extent of the decreased oxygen metabolism.[58] It has been hypothesized that oxygen extraction increases with age, which partly compensates for the observed decrease in the cerebral blood flow. This maintains the oxygen metabolic rate at a higher level than would be expected if oxygen extraction remained constant or decreased with aging.

One concern regarding the accuracy of FDG-PET studies in older patients relates to the effects of age-related brain atrophy on the measurement of cerebral metabolism. The problem is that the resolution of PET causes averaging of signals from the brain tissue and inactive cerebrospinal fluid (CSF) spaces. Therefore, if the subjects have marked atrophy, they will necessarily have a decrease in their mean cerebral metabolism as measured by PET. Several reports that deal with normal aging and brain volume using MR imaging have appeared in the literature.[59,60] Tanna and colleagues[61] measured absolute ventricular and sulcal volumes in healthy elderly subjects and correlated these volumes with age. The best correlations were seen between age and ventricular volumes and age and total brain volumes. Sulcal volumes correlated less well with age. Gur and colleagues[62] studied the relationship between gender differences and the effect of age on brain atrophy using the same methodology. Healthy males had larger brain and CSF volumes compared with age-matched females. Age correlated with decreasing brain volume and increasing CSF volume with steeper regression slopes in males compared with females, suggesting more atrophy with age in males. The greatest degree of atrophy in elderly men occurred in the left hemispheres, whereas women had symmetric changes.

Because brain atrophy might account for a reduction in cerebral metabolism, it has been suggested that changes in brain volume need to be accounted for when considering the results from PET.[63,64] Although atrophy correction of cerebral metabolism has been performed in patients with Alzheimer disease and other types of neurodegenerative diseases, there have been only a limited number of studies performed in normal aging. An early study

measuring cerebral blood volume and oxygen metabolism demonstrated substantial increases in normal-aged individuals compared with younger controls after atrophy correction.[65] The results showed that there were no differences between elderly and younger controls after atrophy correction. A study by Yanase and colleagues[66] using statistical parametric mapping (SPM) analysis showed that although aging resulted in decreased metabolism in the perisylvian and medial frontal regions, these decreases were primarily accounted for by atrophy correction. Other changes were also largely accounted for by atrophy correction.

Yoshii and colleagues[46] used a large number of healthy volunteers to determine the effects of gender, age, brain volume, and cerebrovascular risk factors on CMRGlc values as determined by FDG-PET. When brain atrophy was not considered, mean CMRGlc values were lower in older patients, particularly in the frontal, parietal, and temporal regions. Also, women had significantly higher mean CMRGlc than men. When covariate analysis was used to account for brain atrophy, because brain volume was highly correlated with age, the effects of age and gender on CMRGlc were no longer significant. Cerebrovascular risk factors in this population did not have any effect on CMRGlc. Although important for normalization, statistically, brain atrophy accounted for only 21% of the variance in the CMRGlc.

NEUROTRANSMITTER FUNCTION IN NORMAL AGING

In addition to measuring changes in the cerebral blood flow and metabolism with age, PET can measure neurotransmitter activity, which also changes with age. A large number of neurotransmitter systems can be studied using PET. However, there have been only a limited number of reports using neurotransmitter analogs in the study of the aging brain.

The nigrostriatal dopaminergic pathways have been studied with PET imaging. This pathway is important with regard to extrapyramidal symptoms that occur in the elderly. This system also has particular significance in the study of Parkinson disease. Early in vitro studies generally showed decreases in both D_2 dopamine receptor levels with age.[67–69] Neuroimaging studies measuring D_1 receptor numbers have found inconsistent results, with some suggesting a decrease, some no change, and some an increase with age. However, another study demonstrated significant declines of approximately 7% in D_1 receptor binding every decade in the striatum and several cortical areas.[70]

Several PET studies have shown that the uptake of [18F] fluorodopa (FD), a dopamine precursor in presynaptic neurons, decreases with age (**Fig. 6**). Cordes and colleagues[71] found a 21% decrease in the FD uptake when comparing the uptake in grandparents (ages range from 70–80 years) with that in their grandchildren (ages range from 18–29 years). This study corroborates earlier studies by the same group that indicated similar decreases in FD uptake.[72,73] Further, the authors suggested that this decrease is consistent with the decline in the number of nigral dopaminergic neurons with age. In fact, the average decrease per year of 0.35% in FD uptake is similar to the mean decrease in nigral neurons of 0.6% per year.[74,75] Several other studies have found similar results in both men and women, with age-related decreases in binding of the D_2 dopamine receptor.[76,77] Earlier studies did not find such a decrease in FD uptake with age.[78,79] This inconsistency may be related to the small number of subjects in each study and how regions of interest (ROIs) were drawn. For example, in a related study, ROIs that span the entire striatum showed a relationship of FD uptake with age, whereas small ROIs did not yield the same correlation.[80] Several PET studies using a different radiopharmaceutical, [11C]raclopride that binds D_2 receptors, found a decrease in the receptor density.[81–83] After 30 years of age, there was a 0.6% decline per year in raclopride binding. Another study also demonstrated that the decrease with age in D_2 receptor binding occurs not only in the striatum but also in the extrastriatal regions.[84] D_1 receptor density has also been found to decrease with age using PET imaging.[85]

Radioligands that can measure the dopamine transporter system that removes dopamine from the neuronal synapse into the terminal for storage have also been developed. One PET study by Tedroff and colleagues[86] showed a decline with age of the dopamine transporter using [11C]nomifensine. A more recent study using fluorinated N-3-fluoropropyl-2-beta-carboxymethoxy-3-beta-(4-iodophenyl) nortropane in normal subjects showed a significant age-related decline in caudate and putamen, corresponding to approximately a 7% decline per decade.[87]

The serotonergic system is critical for several functions in the brain and is most notably involved in the regulation of mood. Several studies have examined the changes of the serotonin system with age. For example, a study of serotonin reuptake receptors demonstrated a decline in binding of 9.6% per decade in the thalamus and 10.5% per decade in the midbrain.[88] Another study demonstrated in women a slightly lower rate of decline with age.[89] An age-related decreased activity for the serotonin 1A receptor has been reported with a decline of approximately 10% per decade in several cortical areas except for the medial temporal cortex.[90] However, another report suggested that this finding is more prominent in men and not significant in women.[91] Similar decreases have been reported for the serotonin 2A receptor, with an overall decline of 42% between 23 and 60 years.[92] A more recent study has reported a nonlinear decrease with age in the activity in the serotonin 2A receptor, with most of the decrease occurring through mid-life.[93] The decrease in serotonin 2A receptor binding remains significant even when corrected for age-related cerebral atrophy.[94]

Other neurotransmitter systems have not been widely studied with regard to the effects of aging. One PET study of benzodiazepine receptors demonstrated no significant decline in a small sample of subjects. Several PET studies of the muscarinic cholinergic receptor ligand in 18- to 82-year-old healthy volunteers demonstrated a decrease of 45% to 50% over the age range.[95–97] One study reported increased monoamine oxidase activity with increasing age.[98]

Given the list of radioligands available for PET imaging, it seems that PET may have vast applications in the study of the neurotransmitter effects that result from normal aging as well as neurologic and psychiatric disorders. Several studies have been mentioned earlier, but there remains a significant amount of neurotransmitter systems that are yet to be thoroughly explored with regard to the effects of aging.

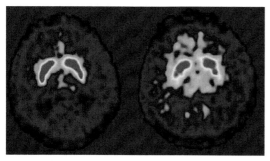

Fig. 6. FDOPA scan in a 50-year-old (*left*) and a 77-year-old (*right*) individual showing decreased uptake in the basal ganglia with aging. FDOPA, fluorodopamine.

OTHER BIOCHEMICAL CHANGES IN NORMAL AGING
Amino Acid Transport

Neutral amino acids (NAAs) are transported across the blood-brain barrier (BBB) via a competitive carrier system. Using positron-emitting labeled NAA analogs, investigators have been able to measure the NAA transport across the BBB with PET imaging.

PET imaging with [^{11}C] L-methionine in pediatric patients showed increased transfer of amino acid across the BBB compared with that in adults.[99] This finding suggests that during developmental periods, the brain allows for a greater influx of amino acids. This finding also suggests that PET might be useful in the study of various inborn errors of metabolism. O'Tuama and colleagues[100] used [^{11}C] L-methionine in adults to study amino acid transport changes with normal aging. They found a decrease in amino acid transport with increasing age, with the frontal lobes particularly affected.[99] The labeling of natural amino acids with positron-emitting isotopes has been found to reduce the accuracy of the kinetic rate constants determined using these compounds. Koeppe and colleagues[101] found no significant decrease in the uptake of the synthetic amino acid [^{11}C]-aminocyclohexanecarboxylate (ACHC). This may more accurately reflect amino acid transport because ACHC is not metabolized in the brain and allows for the simplification of kinetic models. A PET study by Ito and colleagues[102] using L-(2-^{18}F)-fluorophenylalanine (^{18}F-Phe) corroborated the findings with ACHC such that there was no observed decrease in amino acid uptake in the brain with increasing age. They found the increase with aging in the rate constant for the transport of ^{18}F-Phe from the brain to the blood. This may indicate decreased competition between ^{18}F-Phe and natural amino acids because of decreased concentration of intracellular amino acids.

SUMMARY

Functional imaging using SPECT and PET have provided detailed in vivo measurements of cerebral biochemical activity that occur in the normal brain. Functional neuroimaging may also be able to measure the effects of various pharmacologic and nonpharmacologic approaches to prevent the complications associated with normal aging. The ability to interpret findings depends both on technical issues that may affect the "normal" pattern of activity and on "normal" age-related changes. Because such changes can be reflected in cerebral blood flow, glucose and oxygen metabolism, neurotransmitter concentrations, and amino acid metabolism, it is imperative that a complete delineation of the normal range of values and normal variations in measures is performed to adequately evaluate scan findings. Furthermore, the normal variation of functional neuroimaging scans is critical for both clinical and research applications so that appropriate diagnoses may be made and correct interpretation of research findings can be established.

REFERENCES

1. Kuhl DE, Edwards RQ. Image separation of radio-isotope scanning. Radiology 1963;80:653–62.
2. Kuhl DE, Edwards RQ, Ricci AR, et al. The MARK IV system for radionuclide computed tomography of the brain. Radiology 1976;121:405–13.
3. Alavi A, Hirsch LJ. Studies of central nervous system disorders with single photon emission computed tomography and positron emission tomography. Evolution over the past 2 decades. Semin Nucl Med 1991;21:58–81.
4. Diksic M, Reba RC, editors. Radiopharmaceuticals and brain pathology studied with PET and SPECT. Boca Raton (FL): CRC Press; 1991.
5. Kung HF. Overview of radiopharmaceuticals for diagnosis of central nervous disorders. Crit Rev Clin Lab Sci 1991;28:269–86.
6. Ido T, Wan CN, Casella V, et al. Labeled 2-deoxy-glucose analogs. 18F-labeled 2-deoxyglucose-2-fluoro-D-glucose, 2-deoxy-2-fluoro-D-manose and 14C-2-deoxy-2-fluoro-D-glucose. J Label Comp Radiopharm 1978;14:175–83.
7. Ter-Pogossian MM, Phelps ME, Hoffman EJ, et al. A positron emission transaxial tomography for nuclear medicine imaging (PET). Radiology 1975;114:89–98.
8. Phelps ME, Hoffman EJ, Mullani NA, et al. Design considerations for a positron emission transaxial tomograph (PET-III). IEEE Trans Nucl Sci NS 1976;23:516–22.
9. Alavi A, Surti KS, Newberg A. Preliminary report of performance of high resolution gadalinium orthosilicate (GSO)-based dedicated brain PET scanner. J Nucl Med 2002;29:296P.
10. Newberg A, Alavi A, Reivich M. Determination of regional cerebral function with FDG-PET imaging in neuropsychiatric disorders. Semin Nucl Med 2002;32:13–34.
11. Newberg AB, Alavi A, Payer F. Single photon emission computed tomography in Alzheimer's disease and related disorders. Neuroimaging Clin N Am 1995;5(1):103–23.
12. Catafau AM, Parellada E, Lomena F, et al. Baseline, visual deprivation and visual stimulation 99TCm-HMPAO-related changes in visual cortex can be

detected with a single-head SPET system. Nucl Med Commun 1996;17:480–4.

13. Mazziotta JC, Phelps ME. Human sensory stimulation and deprivation: positron emission tomographic results and strategies. Ann Neurol 1984; 15(Suppl):S50–60.

14. Beer J, Blakemore C, Previc FH, et al. Areas of the human brain activated by ambient visual motion, indicating three kinds of self-movement. Exp Brain Res 2002;143:78–88.

15. Castelli F, Happe F, Frith U, et al. Movement and mind: a functional imaging study of perception and interpretation of complex intentional movement patterns. Neuroimage 2000;12(3):314–25.

16. Mirz F, Ovesen T, Ishizu K, et al. Stimulus-dependent central processing of auditory stimuli: a PET study. Scand Audiol 1999;28:161–9.

17. Halpern AR, Zatorre RJ. When that tune runs through your head: a PET investigation of auditory imagery for familiar melodies. Cereb Cortex 1999; 9:697–704.

18. Greene JD, Sommerville RB, Nystrom LE, et al. An fMRI investigation of emotional engagement in moral judgment. Science 2001;293:2105–8.

19. Coull JT, Frith CD. Differential activation of right superior parietal cortex and intraparietal sulcus by spatial and nonspatial attention. Neuroimage 1998;8:176–87.

20. Herzog H, Lele VR, Kuwert T, et al. Changed pattern of regional glucose metabolism during yoga meditative relaxation. Neuropsychobiology 1990–1991;23(4):182–7.

21. Pardo JV, Fox PT, Raichle ME. Localization of a human system for sustained attention by positron emission tomography. Nature 1991;349:61–4.

22. Vogt BA, Finch DM, Olson CR. Functional heterogeneity in cingulate cortex: the anterior executive and posterior evaluative regions. Cereb Cortex 1992;2:435–43.

23. Reiman EM, Lane RD, Ahern GL, et al. Neuroanatomical correlates of externally and internally generated human emotion. Am J Psychiatry 1997; 154:918–25.

24. Phan KL, Wager T, Taylor SF, et al. Functional neuroanatomy of emotion: a meta-analysis of emotion activation studies in PET and fMRI. Neuroimage 2002;16:331–48.

25. Liberzon I, Zubieta JK, Fig LM, et al. mu-Opioid receptors and limbic responses to aversive emotional stimuli. Proc Natl Acad Sci U S A 2002; 99:7084–9.

26. Booij J, Habraken JB, Bergmans P, et al. Imaging of dopamine transporters with iodine-123-FP-CIT SPECT in healthy controls and patients with Parkinson's disease. J Nucl Med 1998;39:1879–84.

27. Ichise M, Ballinger JR, Vines D, et al. Simplified quantification and reproducibility studies of dopamine

28. Chugani HT. Functional brain imaging in pediatrics. Pediatr Clin North Am 1992;39:777–99.

29. Altman DI, Volpe JJ. Positron emission tomography in newborn infants. Clin Perinatol 1991;18:549–62.

30. Chugani HT, Phelps ME, Mazziotta JC. Positron emission tomography study of human brain functional development. Ann Neurol 1987;22:487.

31. Chugani HT, Phelps ME. Maturational changes in cerebral function in infants determined by [18]FDG positron emission tomography. Science 1986;231:840.

32. Takahashi T, Shirane R, Sato S, et al. Developmental changes of cerebral blood flow and oxygen metabolism in children. AJNR Am J Neuroradiol 1999;20:917–22.

33. Kennedy C, Sokoloff L. An adaptation of the nitrous oxide method to the study of the cerebral circulation in children; normal values for cerebral blood flow and cerebral metabolic rate in childhood. J Clin Invest 1957;36:1130.

34. Krausz Y, Bonne O, Gorfine M, et al. Age-related changes in brain perfusion of normal subjects detected by 99mTc-HMPAO SPECT. Neuroradiology 1998;40:428–34.

35. Liu HG, Mountz JM, Inampudi C, et al. A semiquantitative cortical circumferential normalization method for clinical evaluation of rCBF brain SPECT. Clin Nucl Med 1997;22:596–604.

36. Leenders KL, Perani D, Lammertsma AA, et al. Cerebral blood flow, blood volume, and oxygen utilization – normal values and effects of age. Brain 1990;113:27–47.

37. Mozley PD, Sadek AM, Alavi A, et al. Effects of aging on the cerebral distribution of technetium-99m hexamethylpropylene amine oxime in healthy humans. Eur J Nucl Med 1997;24:754–61.

38. Pantano P, Baron JC, Lebrun-Grandie P, et al. Regional cerebral blood flow and oxygen consumption in human aging. Stroke 1984;15:635–41.

39. Martin AJ, Friston KJ, Colebatch JG, et al. Decreases in regional cerebral blood flow with normal aging. J Cereb Blood Flow Metab 1991; 11:684–9.

40. Takada H, Nagata K, Hirata Y, et al. Age-related decline of cerebral oxygen metabolism in normal population detected with positron emission tomography. Neurol Res 1992;14:128–31.

41. Pagani M, Salmaso D, Jonsson C, et al. Regional cerebral blood flow as assessed by principal component analysis and (99m)Tc-HMPAO SPET in healthy subjects at rest: normal distribution and effect of age and gender. Eur J Nucl Med Mol Imaging 2002;29:67–75.

42. Chawluk JB, Alavi A, Hurtig H, et al. Altered patterns of regional cerebral glucose metabolism

in aging and dementia. J Cereb Blood Flow Metab 1985;5:S121–2.

43. deLeon M, George A, Tomanelli J, et al. Positron emission tomography studies of normal aging, a replication of PET III and 18-FDG using PET IV and II-CDG. Neurobiol Aging 1987;8:319–23.

44. Chawluk JB, Alavi A, Dann R, et al. Positron emission tomography in aging and dementia. Effect of cerebral atrophy. J Nucl Med 1987;28:431–7.

45. Weiss D, Souder E, Alavi A, et al. Effects of normal aging on whole brain and regional glucose metabolism as assessed by F-18 positron emission tomography. J Nucl Med 1990;31:771.

46. Yoshii F, Barker WW, Chang JY, et al. Sensitivity of cerebral glucose metabolism to age, gender, brain volume, brain atrophy, and cerebrovascular risk factors. J Cereb Blood Flow Metab 1988;8:654–61.

47. Kuhl DE, Metter EJ, Riege WH, et al. Effects of human aging on patterns of local cerebral glucose utilization determined by the 18-F fluorodeoxyglucose method. J Cereb Blood Flow Metab 1982;2:163–71.

48. Alavi A, Jolles PR, Jamieson DG, et al. Anatomic and functional changes of the brain in normal aging and dementia as demonstrated by MRI, CT, and PET. Nucl Med Ann 1989;49–79.

49. Loessner A, Alavi A, Lewandrowski KU, et al. Regional cerebral function determined by FDG-PET in healthy volunteers: normal patterns and changes with age. J Nucl Med 1995;36:1141–9.

50. Eberling JL, Nordahl TE, Kusubov N, et al. Reduced temporal lobe glucose metabolism in aging. J Neuroimaging 1995;5:178–82.

51. Alavi A, Chawluck JB, Hurtig H, et al. Determination of patterns of regional cerebral glucose metabolism in normal aging and dementia. J Nucl Med 1985;26:P69.

52. Miura SA, Shapiro MB, Grady CL, et al. Effects of gender on glucose utilization rates in healthy humans: a positron emission tomography study. J Neurosci Res 1990;27:500–4.

53. Kawachi T, Ishii K, Sakamoto S, et al. Gender differences in cerebral glucose metabolism: a PET study. J Neurol Sci 2002;199:79–83.

54. Kuhl DE, Metter EJ, Riege WH, et al. The effect of normal aging on patterns of local cerebral glucose utilization. Ann Neurol 1984;15(Suppl):S133–7.

55. Hawkins RA, Mazziotta JC, Phelps ME, et al. Cerebral glucose metabolism as a function of age in man: influence of the rate constants in fluorodeoxyglucose. J Cereb Blood Flow Metab 1983;3:250–3.

56. Dastur DK. Cerebral blood flow and metabolism in normal human aging, pathological aging, and senile dementia. J Cereb Blood Flow Metab 1985; 5:1.

57. Yamaguchi T, Kanno I, Nemura K, et al. Reduction in regional cerebral metabolic rate of oxygen during human aging. Stroke 1986;17:1220.

58. Frackowiak RSJ, Gibbs JM. Cerebral metabolism and blood flow in normal aging and pathological aging. In: Pagistretti PL, editor. Functional radionuclide imaging of the brain. New York: Raven Press; 1983.

59. Wahlund LO, Agartz I, Almqvist O, et al. The brain in healthy aged individuals. MR imaging. Radiology 1990;174:675–9.

60. Jernigan TL, Archibald SL, Berhow MT, et al. Cerebral structure on MRI, Part I: localization of age-related changes. Biol Psychiatry 1991;29:55–67.

61. Tanna NK, Kohn MI, Horwich DN, et al. Analysis of brain and cerebrospinal fluid volumes with MR imaging. Impact on PET data, correction for atrophy. Radiology 1991;178:123–30.

62. Gur RC, Mozley PD, Resnick SM, et al. Gender differences in age effect on brain atrophy measured by magnetic resonance imaging. Proc Natl Acad Sci 1991;88:2845–9.

63. Clark C, Hayden M, Hollenberg S, et al. Controlling for cerebral atrophy in positron emission tomography data. J Cereb Blood Flow Metab 1987;7: 510–2.

64. Schlageter NL, Horwitz B, Creasey H, et al. Relation of measured brain glucose utilization and cerebral atrophy in man. J Neurol Neurosurg Psychiatr 1987;50:779–85.

65. Herscovitch P, Auchus AP, Gado M, et al. Correction of positron emission tomography data for cerebral atrophy. J Cereb Blood Flow Metab 1986;6(1): 120–4.

66. Yanase D, Matsunari I, Yajima K, et al. Brain FDG PET study of normal aging in Japanese: effect of atrophy correction. Eur J Nucl Med Mol Imaging 2005;32(7):794–805.

67. Rinne JO, Lonnberg P, Marjamaki P. Age-dependent decline in human brain dopamine D1 and D2 response. Brain Res 1990;508:349–52.

68. Rinne JO. Muscarinic and dopaminergic receptors in the aging human brain. Brain Res 1987; 404:162–8.

69. Morgan DG, Marcusson JO, Nyberg P, et al. Divergent changes in D1 and D2 dopamine binding sites in human brain during aging. Neurobiol Aging 1987;8:195–201.

70. Wang Y, Chan GL, Holden JE, et al. Age-dependent decline of dopamine D1 receptors in human brain: a PET study. Synapse 1998;30:56–61.

71. Cordes M, Snow BJ, Cooper S, et al. Age-dependent decline of nigrostriatal dopaminergic function: a positron emission tomographic study of grandparents and their grandchildren. Ann Neurol 1994;36:667–70.

72. Bhatt MH, Snow BJ, Martin WRW, et al. Positron emission tomography suggests that the rate of progression of idiopathic parkinsonism is slow. Ann Neurol 1991;29:673–7.

73. Martin WRW, Palmer MR, Patlak CS, et al. Nigrostriatal function in man studied with positron emission tomography. Ann Neurol 1989;26:535–42.

74. McGeer PL, McGeer EG, Suzuki JS. Aging and extrapyramidal function. Arch Neurol 1977;34:33–5.

75. Gibb WRG, Lees AJ. Anatomy, pigmentation, ventral and dorsal subpopulations of the substantia nigra, and differential cell death in Parkinson's disease. J Neurol Neurosurg Psychiatr 1991;54:388–96.

76. Inoue M, Suhara T, Sudo Y, et al. Age-related reduction of extrastriatal dopamine D2 receptor measured by PET. Life Sci 2001;69:1079–84.

77. Kaasinen V, Kemppainen N, Nagren K, et al. Age-related loss of extrastriatal dopamine D(2) -like receptors in women. J Neurochem 2002;81:1005–10.

78. Sawle GV, Colebatch JG, Shah A, et al. Striatal function in normal aging: implications for Parkinson's disease. Ann Neurol 1990;28:799–804.

79. Eidelberg D, Takikawa S, Dhawan V, et al. Striatal [^{18}F]-DOPA uptake: absence of an aging effect. J Cereb Blood Flow Metab 1993;13:881–8.

80. Vingerhoets FJG, Snow BJ, Schulzer MJ, et al. Reproducibility of fluorine-18-6-fluorodopa positron emission tomography in normal human subjects. J Nucl Med 1994;35:18–24.

81. Rinne JO, Hietala J, Ruotsalainen U, et al. Decrease in human striata dopamine D2 receptor density with age: a PET study with [^{11}C] raclopride. J Cereb Blood Flow Metab 1993;13:310–4.

82. Volkow ND, Wang GJ, Fowler JS, et al. Measuring age-related changes in dopamine D2 receptors with 11C-raclopride and ^{18}F-N-methylspiroperidol. Psychiatry Res 1996;67:11–6.

83. Antonini A, Leenders KL. Dopamine D2 receptors in normal human brain: effect of age measured by positron emission tomography (PET) and [^{11}C] raclopride. Ann NY Acad Sci 1993;695:81–5.

84. Kaasinen V, Vilkman H, Hietala J, et al. Age-related dopamine D2/D3 receptor loss in extrastriatal regions of the human brain. Neurobiol Aging 2000;21:683–8.

85. Suhara T, Fukuda H, Inoue O, et al. Age-related changes in human D1 dopamine receptors measured by positron emission tomography. Psychopharmacology 1991;103:41–5.

86. Tedroff J, Aquilonius SM, Hartvig P, et al. Monoamine re-uptake sites in the human brain evaluated in vivo by means of [^{11}C] nomifensine and positron emission tomography: the effects of age and Parkinson's disease. Acta Neurol Scand 1988;77: 192–201.

87. Kazumata K, Dhawan V, Chaly T, et al. Dopamine transporter imaging with fluorine-18-FPCIT and PET. J Nucl Med 1998;39(9):1521–30.

88. Yamamoto M, Suhara T, Okubo Y, et al. Age-related decline of serotonin transporters in living human brain of healthy males. Life Sci 2002;71:751–7.

89. Kuikka JT, Tammela L, Bergstrom KA, et al. Effects of ageing on serotonin transporters in healthy females. Eur J Nucl Med 2001;28:911–3.

90. Tauscher J, Verhoeff NP, Christensen BK, et al. Serotonin 5-HT1A receptor binding potential declines with age as measured by [^{11}C]WAY-100635 and PET. Neuropsychopharmacology 2001;24:522–30.

91. Meltzer C, Drevets WC, Price JC, et al. Gender-specific aging effects on the serotonin 1A receptor. Brain Res 2001;895:9–17.

92. Baeken C, D'haenen H, Flamen P, et al. 123I-5-I-R91150, a new single-photon emission tomography ligand for 5-HT2A receptors: influence of age and gender in healthy subjects. Eur J Nucl Med 1998;25:1617–22.

93. Sheline YI, Mintun MA, Moerlein SM, et al. Greater loss of 5-HT(2A) receptors in midlife than in late life. Am J Psychiatry 2002;159:430–5.

94. Meltzer CC, Smith G, Price JC, et al. Reduced binding of [^{18}F]altanserin to serotonin type 2A receptors in aging: persistence of effect after partial volume correction. Brain Res 1998;813:167–71.

95. Suhara T, Inoue O, Kobayashi K, et al. Age-related changes in human muscarinic acetylcholine receptors measured by positron emission tomography. Neurosci Lett 1993;149:225–8.

96. Lee KS, Frey KA, Koeppe RA, et al. In vivo quantification of cerebral muscarinic receptors in normal human aging using positron emission tomography and [^{11}C]tropanyl benzilate. J Cereb Blood Flow Metab 1996;16:303–10.

97. Dewey SL, Volkow ND, Logan J, et al. Age-related decreases in muscarinic cholinergic receptor binding in the human brain measured with positron emission tomography (PET). J Neurosci Res 1990; 27:569–75.

98. Fowler JS, Volkow ND, Wang GJ, et al. Age-related increases in brain monoamine oxidase B in living healthy human subjects. Neurobiol Aging 1997; 18:431–5.

99. O'Tuama LA, Phillips PC, Smith QR, et al. L-Methionine uptake by human cerebral cortex. Maturation from infancy to old age. J Nucl Med 1991;32:16.

100. O'Tuama LA, Guilarte TR, Douglass KH, et al. Assessment of [^{11}C]-L-methionine transport into the human brain. J Cereb Blood Flow Metab 1988;8:341–5.

101. Koeppe RA, Mangner T, Betz AL, et al. Use of [^{11}C] aminocyclohexane-carboxylate for the measurement of amino acid uptake and distribution volume in human brain. J Cereb Blood Flow Metab 1990; 10:727–39.

102. Ito H, Hatazawa J, Murakami M, et al. Aging effect on neutral amino acid transport at the blood-brain barrier measured with L-[2-^{18}F]-Fluorophenylalanine and PET. J Nucl Med 1995;35:1232–7.

Evaluation of Early Dementia (Mild Cognitive Impairment)

R.S. Osorio, MD[a,b,c], V. Berti, MD[a,d], L. Mosconi, PhD[a],
Y. Li, MD[a], L. Glodzik, MD, PhD[a], S. De Santi, PhD[a],
M.J. de Leon, EdD[a,e],*

KEYWORDS

- PET scan • Dementia • Mild cognitive impairment
- Early diagnosis

Alzheimer disease (AD) is the leading cause of dementia in the elderly, accounting for up to 70% of dementia cases, and is the sixth leading cause of death in the United States.[1] The provisional diagnosis of AD is based on clinical history, neurologic examination, cognitive testing, and neuroimaging, whereas the definitive diagnosis of AD is based on the postmortem observation of specific pathologic lesions; intracellular neurofibrillary tangles (NFTs); amyloid beta (Aβ) deposition in the form of senile plaques in the extracellular spaces and in blood vessels; and neuronal and synaptic losses, resulting in clinically detectable brain atrophy in known vulnerable brain areas.[2–4]

Patients with very early cognitive symptoms constitute a biologically heterogeneous population, clinically difficult to distinguish from those with known physiologic changes associated with aging, functional disturbances of depression, and drug-induced or metabolic or vitamin deficiency states. Clinically, an intermediate stage has been described using various discrete categories, such as mild cognitive impairment (MCI), cognitive impairment not demented,[5] prodromal AD,[6] and questionable dementia,[7] among others.[8–10] These terms are not specific for AD, but they have in common that they refer to nondemented persons with cognitive deficits, representing a clinical syndrome that has been shown to have a high risk of progressing to a dementia and AD.

Consensus criteria have been recently formulated by the International Working Group on Mild Cognitive Impairment[11] to unify these terminologies (**Box 1**). The term MCI, originally defined by Reisberg and colleagues,[8] describes a pre-AD syndrome. Petersen and colleagues[12] have further elaborated the term MCI and observed that annually 10% to 15% convert to AD.[13,14] However, some MCIs remain stable or even improve spontaneously.[15] Three subtypes have been suggested on the basis of single or multiple cognitive

Supported by a grant from the Alzheimer's Disease Research Unit. CIEN Foundation-Reina Sofia Foundation, Carlos III Institute of Health.

[a] Department of Psychiatry, Center for Brain Health, Silberstein Alzheimer's Institute, Center of Excellence on Brain Aging, NYU Langone Medical Center, 145 East 32nd Street, 5th Floor, New York, NY 10016, USA

[b] Department of Pathology and Psychiatry, Alzheimer's Disease Center, Silberstein Alzheimer's Institute, Center of Excellence on Brain Aging, NYU Langone Medical Center, 145 East 32nd Street, 2nd Floor, New York, NY 10016, USA

[c] Alzheimer's Disease Research Unit, CIEN Foundation-Reina Sofia Foundation, Carlos III Institute of Health, Valderrebollo 5, (Complejo Alzheimer), PAU de Vallecas, Madrid 28031, Spain

[d] Department of Clinical Pathophysiology, Nuclear Medicine Unit, University of Florence, Viale Morgagni 85, Florence 50134, Italy

[e] Nathan Kline Institute, 140 Old Orangeburg Road, Orangeburg, NY 10962, USA

* Corresponding author. Department of Psychiatry, Center for Brain Health, Silberstein Alzheimer's Institute, Center of Excellence on Brain Aging, NYU Langone Medical Center, 145 East 32nd Street, 5th Floor, New York, NY 10016.

E-mail address: Mony.DeLeon@nyumc.org

Box 1
Consensus criteria for MCI

- The individual is neither normal nor demented.
- There is evidence of cognitive deterioration, shown either by objectively measured decline over time or by subjective report of decline by self or informant in conjunction with objective cognitive deficits.
- Activities of daily life are preserved, and complex instrumental functions are either intact or minimally impaired.

Data from Winblad B, Palmer K, Kivipelto M, et al. Mild cognitive impairment—beyond controversies, towards a consensus: report of the International Working Group on Mild Cognitive Impairment. J Intern Med 2004;256(3):240–6.

deficits[11]: amnestic MCI (aMCI), multiple-domain MCI (amnestic or nonamnestic), and single non-memory domain MCI. The aMCI subtype more likely represents a prodromal form of AD,[10] whereas patients with nonamnestic MCI may have a higher likelihood of progressing to atypical AD[16] or other dementia syndromes, such as vascular dementia (VD), frontotemporal lobar degeneration (FTLD), or Lewy body dementia (LBD).[15,17]

Several pathology studies have shown that the lesions of AD are found in normal elderly subjects,[2,3] possibly heralding a transitional pathologic period between normal aging and cognitive symptoms. The studies that have investigated the neuropathology of MCI also show evidence of significant neuropathologic and neurobiologic changes that are qualitatively similar to those observed in the brains of subjects with frank AD-like dementia.[18,19] These findings highlight the need and potential to identify individuals at an earlier point in their cognitive decline, where therapeutic interventions could be more effective. For this purpose, some investigators have proposed strategies to study patients with AD in early stages, analyzing minimally impaired subjects with subjective memory complaints (SMC)[19,20] or presymptomatic cognitively normal individuals with known risk factors for developing late-onset AD. These approaches, however, suffer the same uncertainties as the MCI label by including other predementia syndromes and psychiatric comorbidities.[11,13,21]

In light of the difficulties to find an appropriate early-dementia profile, there is now a general tendency to shift from a symptomatic and categorical characterization of early AD to a more biologic and dimensional approach based on biomarkers,

imaging, prospective studies, and neuropathology.[22] PET tracers are sensitive to the earliest biologic changes that are found in AD (neuronal and synapse loss, NFT, Aβ plaques), can be studied longitudinally, and are increasingly consistent with the known histology of the disease in the few cases that have been studied postmortem after neuroimaging.[23–25] PET imaging therefore, can help, to some degree, to overcome the clinical difficulties of the early detection of AD and to improve the diagnostic accuracy by using it as a diagnostic tool to discriminate among normal aging and early AD; as a prognostic tool in longitudinal studies to predict conversion to MCI or AD; or as a presymptomatic biomarker in cognitively normal individuals to identify persons at higher risk for future symptoms. This article focuses on these recent PET studies in the presymptomatic and preclinical stages of late-onset AD and discusses its use in clinical settings.

FDG-PET STUDIES

[^{18}F] 2-fluoro-2-deoxy-D-glucose (FDG)–PET has long been used to track AD-related brain changes by providing qualitative and quantitative estimates of the cerebral metabolic rate of glucose (CMRglc).[26] FDG uptake in the brain reflects local glucose consumption[27] and can be interpreted as an index of synaptic functioning and density.[28] Synaptic dysfunction and neuronal degeneration regularly lead to a decline of CMRglc in the affected parts of the brain and in regions that receive projections from these primary diseased neurons.[22,29,30] In the early stages of AD, the most prominent and consistent CMRglc findings are decreased metabolism found in the parieto-temporal areas, precuneus, posterior cingulate cortex (PCC), and (as more recently reported) entorhinal cortex (EC)[31] and hippocampus (Hip).[32] As the disease progresses, frontal association cortices become involved, whereas cerebellum, striatum, primary visual, and sensorimotor cortices remain preserved.[22,33,34] The topography of involvement is consistent with the progression of NFT pathology delineated by Braak and Braak[2] but not with the time course of the expansion of Aβ pathology in the brain.[4] FDG-PET studies in normal aging show CMRglc reductions in the frontal and anterior cingulate cortex (ACC), accompanied by small reductions in global CMRglc.[30,35]

FDG-PET Diagnosis of MCI

So far, no specific CMRglc pattern has been recognized to be a hallmark for MCI,[22,36] probably because of the already described heterogeneity of the construct. Recent FDG-PET studies that have focused on aMCI show a more characteristic hypometabolism pattern in some of the brain regions typically affected in clinical AD, such as PCC, parietotemporal cortices, and medial temporal lobe (MTL), although the magnitude of the reductions is milder than that in clinical patients with AD.[33,36–40]

In a recent multicenter study[41] that examined different MCI subgroups, 70% of patients with aMCI demonstrated a pattern of hypometabolism restricted to PCC and Hip. The remaining 30% showed wider CMRglc abnormalities, involving parietotemporal cortex, PCC, and MTL, which were observed also in most MCI patients with deficits in multiple cognitive domains, frequently with additional frontal hypometabolism. These data also suggest that the extent of hypometabolism may correlate with the severity of cognitive impairment, considering single domain aMCI as an initial AD stage and multiple-domain MCI as a more advanced stage of the disease as it has already been described in MCI clinical longitudinal conversion studies.[42] Other studies have shown a more variable metabolic profile in patients with nonamnestic MCI, ranging from isolated Hip CMRglc reductions to metabolic patterns consistent with different types of dementia, such as AD, FTLD, and LBD.[31,32,41,43–45]

Prediction of Decline from Normal Cognition to MCI and to AD

In addition to cross-sectional FDG-PET studies focusing on the differentiation of MCI from normal aging, growing bodies of longitudinal FDG-PET reports are examining the predictive value of these measures in predicting the decline among healthy controls (NLs) to MCI and from MCI to AD.

Little work has been done with FDG-PET to monitor the progression from NLs to MCI or AD. Such studies are limited because of the intrinsic difficulty of observing clinical change for a group with a low incidence of decline (1%–3% per year) and a slow progression of cognitive change.[12] Large subject samples and long follow-up intervals are required to observe cognitively normal persons over time, until they develop dementia. Only 3 FDG-PET studies have monitored decline from NLs to MCI and dementia (**Table 1**).[31,46,47] In these 3 studies, reduced baseline CMRglc in the EC,[31] Hip,[47] and left angular and left middle temporal gyri[46] predicted change to MCI or AD or correlated with cognitive decline. Of note, these effects remained significant after correcting the CMRglc values for partial volume effects of atrophy as determined from MRI, suggesting that

these early CMRglc reductions in MCI are in excess of tissue loss and represent a real reduction of glucose consumption per gram in the remaining brain tissue.[31]

More evidence exists for the metabolic changes that predict the decline from MCI to AD (**Table 2**).[37–39,42,48–52] A recent meta-analysis[54] reported that FDG-PET had an average sensitivity of 88.9% and an average specificity of 84.9% in the prediction of the MCI conversion to AD, with prediction accuracies ranging from 75% to 100%.[38,42,48,49,51] Most studies focused on patients with aMCI, and the data show that baseline CMRglc reductions are more pronounced in those with aMCI who later develop the symptoms of AD as compared with those who remain stable. Moreover, there is evidence showing that the metabolic changes in the declining patients with aMCI are progressive and that longitudinal CMRglc measures both predict and correlate who will decline to AD.[38] Several reports demonstrated that the aMCI converters show the typical AD functional pattern, with hypometabolism in the parietotemporal cortex and PCC, compared with the nonconverters.[42,51] Other studies, instead, highlight a more prominent CMRglc impairment in ventromedial prefrontal regions in aMCI converters than in nonconverters.[53] In summary, these FDG-PET studies with clinical follow-up periods provide evidence for a topographical progression of CMRglc abnormalities, which seem to originate in the MTL during the normal stages of cognition, extend to the PCC at the MCI stage of AD, and spread to the parietotemporal cortices in full-blown dementia.[22]

"AT RISK" POPULATIONS
Apolipoprotein E Epsilon 4 Genotype

The epsilon 4 allele of the apolipoprotein E (APOE) gene on chromosome 19 is a widely established genetic risk factor for late-onset AD.[55,56] APOEE4 is specifically thought to maintain neuronal homeostasis by transporting lipids, such as cholesterol and phospholipids, which are responsible for neuronal plasticity, throughout the central nervous system.[57] There are 3 common human APOEE4 isoforms (E2, E3, and E4); the APOEE4 allele operates as a genetic risk modifier for AD by increasing the risk for developing AD and by decreasing the age at onset.[55,56] Several FDG-PET studies have examined the effects of the APOEE4 allele on CMRglc in nondemented individuals, reporting that compared with noncarriers, cognitively normal APOEE4 carriers have similar (but milder) hypometabolism in the same brain regions as those found in patients with aMCI and

Table 1
Longitudinal FDG-PET studies focusing on the decline from normal cognition to MCI or AD

Reference	Subjects	N Conv	Follow-up	Method	PET Findings	Operating Characteristics
de Leon et al,[31] 2001	67 normal elderly (48 completed the study)	11 (22%) to MCI 1 (2%) to AD	3 y	ROI	Reduced CMRglc in the EC. CMRglc reductions were found in the EC, Hip, and LTL during the progression to MCI	Prediction of MCI diagnosis with 83% sensitivity and 85% specificity
Jagust et al,[46] 2006	60 normal elderly (52 completed the study)	5 (8%) to CIND 1 (2%) to AD	3.8 y	SPM	Reduced CMRglc in the left angular and left middle temporal gyri was associated with faster cognitive decline (the 6 converters were excluded)	
Mosconi et al,[47] 2008	77 normal elderly	19 (25%) to MCI 6 (8%) to AD 5 (6%) other dementias	7.2 y	SPM	Reduced CMRglc in Hip	Prediction of progression from NL to AD with 81% accuracy and decline from NL to MCI with 71% accuracy

Data from Winblad B, Palmer K, Kivipelto M, et al. Mild cognitive impairment—beyond controversies, towards a consensus: report of the International Working Group on Mild Cognitive Impairment. J Intern Med 2004;256:240–6.

Table 2
Longitudinal FDG-PET studies focusing on the decline from MCI to AD

Reference	Subjects	N Conv	Follow-up	Method	CMRglc Reductions Conv vs N Conv
Heroltz et al,[48] 1999	MCI	19/52 (36%)	2 y	ROI	Global CMRglc reduction (ratio global/cerebellum)
Arnáiz et al,[49] 2001	MCI	9/20 (45%)	36 mo	ROI	Temporoparietal cortex
Chetelat et al,[37] 2003	aMCI	7/17 (41%)	18 mo	SPM	STG
Silverman et al,[50] 2003	MCI	58/128 (45%)	3 y	NA	Temporoparietal cortex
Drzezga et al,[38] 2003	MCI	8/22 (36%)	1 y	NEUROSTAT	PCC, precuneus
Mosconi et al,[39] 2004	aMCI	8/37 (22%)	12 mo	SPM	IPL
Anchisi et al,[51] 2005	aMCI	14/48 (29%)	12 mo	SPM	IPL, PCC, Hip, PHG
Drzezga et al,[52] 2005	25/30 (83%) mdMCI, 5/30 (17%) aMCI	12/30 (40%)	15 mo	NEUROSTAT	IPL, TC, MTL, PCC, IPFC
Fouquet et al,[53] 2009	aMCI	7/17 (41%)	18 mo	SPM	Ventromedial prefrontal regions (ACC, subgenual area)

Abbreviations: Conv, converters to AD; IPFC, inferior prefrontal cortex; IPL, inferior parietal lobe; mdMCI, multiple-domain MCI; NA, not applicable; nconv, nonconverters to AD; PHG, parahippocampal gyrus; ROI, region of interest analysis of CMRglc; SPM, statistical parametric mapping; STG, superior temporal gyrus; TC, temporal cortex.

AD.[56–62] In particular, the metabolic reductions involve the PCC/precuneus and parietotemporal and frontal areas and are not explained by brain atrophy.[61,63,64] Changes are also observed in 20- to 40-year-old APOEE4 carriers.[61] In a recent study, a hypometabolism by genotype interaction was found in APOEE4 carriers with SMC, such that the most severe CMRglc reductions were found in the E4+/SMC+ with respect to other subgroups. This effect was maximal in the anterior parahippocampal gyrus (region of the EC).[58] Moreover, several studies on middle-aged cognitively normal APOEE4 carriers show that the metabolic reductions are progressive and that they correlate with reductions in cognitive performance.[60,63] In addition, there is evidence that the *APOEE4* allele is associated with an accelerated longitudinal CMRglc decline in healthy elderly converting to MCI (see **Table 1**).[31] Still, it remains unknown whether the cortical CMRglc reductions observed in cognitively normal E4 carriers are predictive of subsequent decline to AD. The authors investigated the ability of FDG-PET to predict AD among patients with MCI after considering the APOEE4 genotype.[38] At baseline, the E4 carriers showed an AD-like metabolic pattern relative to the noncarriers, with the expected CMRglc reductions within the PCC and parietotemporal areas, bilaterally. Besides, the E4 carriers who later converted to AD had additional frontal hypometabolism involving the ACC and inferior frontal cortex. Within the group of nonconverters, the E4 carriers showed PCC and parietotemporal CMRglc reductions relative to the noncarriers. This raises the question as to whether when examining a PET scan from an APOEE4 carrier with hypometabolism, this is a sign of increased risk for AD or only a genetic concomitant with no known clinical implications.

Some investigators[65] have suggested that PET metabolic reduction in E4 carriers is related to disease susceptibility and could be viewed as a presymptomatic neuroimaging endophenotype of AD, but as mentioned earlier, this has not been validated. Endophenotypes are biomarkers that are associated with illness in the population, heritable, state-independent, cosegregate with the illness within families, and found in nonaffected family members at a higher rate than in the general population.[66] This construct could help to evaluate risk modifiers before the onset of the symptoms in these subjects[65] and also help to study heritable or nonheritable protective effects in APOEE4 carriers who do not express the endophenotype.

Maternal Family History of AD

After an advanced age, having a first-degree family history with late-onset AD, especially an affected parent, is the most prominent risk factor for developing AD among cognitively normal subjects.[67] First-degree relatives of patients with AD are at 4- to 10-fold increased risk of developing AD as compared with individuals with no family history.[68–70] Although there is mixed evidence for parent-of-origin effects in late-onset AD families,[71,72] several epidemiologic data indicate that having an AD-affected mother confers greater risk than having an AD-affected father.[71] The authors' recent FDG-PET study on normal individuals with parental family history of AD showed that subjects with a maternal family history of AD exhibited CMRglc reductions as compared with subjects with a paternal history and those without a family history of AD.[73] In particular, as compared with individuals with no family history and those with an AD-affected father, individuals with a maternal history of AD showed CMRglc reductions in parietotemporal and medial temporal cortices, PCC/precuneus, and frontal cortex, which are the typically hypometabolic regions in patients with clinical AD. Moreover, in a 2-year longitudinal FDG-PET study, the authors found that regional CMRglc continues to decline in normal individuals with maternal family history during the follow-up.[74] In particular, in subjects with a maternal family history, the CMRglc declines in the same AD-vulnerable regions that were hypometabolic at baseline, such as the parietotemporal and PCC cortices. CMRglc in these regions was reduced 13% at baseline and 23% at follow-up. The annual rate of decline in subjects with a maternal family AD history was significantly greater (-3.14 ± 1.3 µmol/100 g/min/y) than that observed in subjects without a family history of AD (-0.75 ± 1.5 µmol/100 g/min/y) and those with paternal family history (-0.56 ± 0.91 µmol/100 g/min/y). The biologic and genetic mechanisms that underlie the CMRglc reductions in normal individuals with maternal family history are unknown. Among the possibilities, hypometabolism may be a result of a combination of defective mitochondrial function and possible mitochondrial

DNA mutations,[75] epigenetic imprinting, chromosome X transmission, and mutations in nuclear DNA affecting mitochondrial function. The evidence to date does not suggest a linkage to APOEE4; nevertheless, the PET endophenotype approach used to study APOEE4[65] is being used to clarify the maternal pattern of heritability.

AMYLOID PET IMAGING

Before the development of PET radioligands that could measure Aβ plaques and NFT, these protein deposits could only be observed at autopsy and crudely estimated in CSF samples. To date, several PET tracers have been developed to provide measures of these deposits in vivo. N-Methyl-[11C]-2-(4′-methylaminophenyl)-6-hydroxy-benzothiazole, the best known tracer which is also known as Pittsburgh compound-B (PIB), binds preferably to Aβ plaques and Aβ fibrils[76] and is currently in widespread research use to assess in vivo Aβ burden. Another tracer, 2-(1-(6-[(2-[18F]fluoroethyl)(methyl)amino]-2-naphthyl)ethylidene)malono nitrile (FDDNP), binds to Aβ plaques and NFT,[77,78] although the experience with its use is more limited. Other amyloid imaging agents include 11C-SB13,[79] 11C-BF-227,[80] and 18F-BAY94-9172[81] but are not discussed in this article as limited clinical data are available.

PIB

PIB-PET studies have demonstrated 50% to 90% differences between the brain PIB retention in patients with AD and NLs, with accuracies approaching 90%.[76,81–83] These effects are most evident in the middle and prefrontal cortices, parietotemporal regions, PCC/precuneus, occipital lobes, thalamus, and striatum.[76,82–84] Voxel-based methods for the statistical analysis of PIB retention have confirmed the region of interest (ROI) analysis results.[85] PIB-PET discriminates successfully between AD patients and age-matched NLs. PIB-PET also discriminates between MCI and AD,[85] even though it shows significant PIB retention in the AD range in as many as 61% of MCI[82,83,85] and 22% of NLs.[82] In patients with MCI, PIB uptake shows a bimodal distribution, with a subset having low PIB retention and a subset with high PIB in the AD range,[86] whereas in the NL elderly, PIB binding spans a broad range from amyloid negative to AD levels.[87,88] These bindings are consistent with the known pattern of Aβ plaque deposition observed at postmortem study in AD or aged nondemented patients[2,4] and also correlate with reductions in CSF Aβ1-42[89] and postmortem studies of patients with AD

Table 3
Longitudinal PIB-PET studies focusing on the decline from NC or MCI to AD

References	Tracer	Subjects	N Conv	Follow-up	Method	SE	SP	PET Findings Conv vs N Conv
Small et al,[78] 2006	FDDNP	12 (8 normal elderly, 4 MCI)	3/12 (25%), 1 NL to MCI, 2 MCI to AD	2 y	ROI			3 converters had FDDNP binding increases of between 5.5% and 11.2%
Forsberg et al,[86] 2008	PIB	21 MCI	7/11 (64%) PIB+, 0/10 (0%) PIB−	8 mo	ROI	64%	100%	PIB retention in MCI converters was comparable with that in patients with AD. All converters were PIB+ and aMCI
Koivunen et al,[96] 2008	PIB	15 aMCI, 22 controls	6/13 (46%) PIB+, 0/2 (0%), PIB−	2 y	ROI	46%	100%	All converters had increased PIB uptake in the PCC and frontal cortices
Wolk et al,[88] 2009	PIB	23 MCI	5/13 (38%) PIB+, 0/10 (0%) PIB−	21 mo	ROI	38%	100%	3/30 (30%) of MCI patients with PIB negative scans no longer qualified for this designation (ie, "reversion to normal")
Okello et al,[97] 2009	PIB	31 aMCI (17/14)	14/17 (82%) PIB+, 1/14 (7% of PIB−)	1–3 y	ROI, SPM	82%	93%	Significantly higher PIB binding was detected in the PIB+ faster converters

Abbreviations: Conv, converters to AD; IPFC, inferior prefrontal cortex; IPL, inferior parietal lobe; mdMCI, multiple-domain MCI; nconv, nonconverters to AD; PHG, parahippocampal gyrus; ROI, region of interest analysis of CMRglc; SE, sensitivity; SP, specificity; SPM, statistical parametric mapping; STG, superior temporal gyrus; TC, temporal cortex.

who had undergone PIB-PET imaging before death.[25] PIB negative patients tend to have a - milder cognitive profile[90] and sometimes revert to a normal cognition.[88] However, more studies are needed to clarify the early and relative predictive utility of PIB imaging in assessing the risk for progressive cognitive decline among these patients without significant PIB uptake.

FDDNP

Several FDDNP-PET studies have demonstrated significant retention in AD in the temporal, parietal, PCC, and frontal regions compared with controls.[78,91,92] FDDNP-PET discrimination between AD and MCI is controversial as the 2 studies published to date show discrepant results in terms of FDDNP binding in the MCI group.[78,92] This could be explained by the narrow range of tracer binding across subjects (5%–8% binding increase in patients with MCI and AD relative to controls)[93] or the differences in patient selection.[92] FDDNP binding in patients with MCI seems to be more diffuse and widespread,[92] different from the bimodal distribution (AD-like or NL-like) of patients with MCI in the PIB studies.[88,92]

Prediction of Decline from MCI to AD with Amyloid Tracers

To date, 5 studies[80,88,89,94,95] have analyzed the progression from NL or MCI to AD based on amyloid binding and clinical follow-up periods (**Table 3**). The number of converters (those who declined) in the aMCI PIB positive patients ranged from 38% to 82%, with higher PIB binding in the group of converters, and almost no conversions (0%–7%) in the group with lower PIB binding.[86,97] One follow-up PIB-PET publication indicated small longitudinal progression of PIB retention,[94] suggesting that amyloid deposition may plateau at the AD stage. It is less clear, however, at what stage $A\beta$ deposition, as detectable by PIB-PET, plateaus in any given patient during the clinical transition from MCI to AD.[97] Finally, in the only longitudinal FDDNP results published to date, a total of 12 subjects were observed for 2 years. Nine of these patients, who remained clinically stable (7 controls and 2 patients with MCI), had FDDNP binding increases of less than or equal to 3%. By contrast, 3 patients who showed clinical evidence of disease progression (1 control subject was reclassified as having MCI, and 2 individuals with MCI were reclassified as having AD) had FDDNP binding increases of between 5.5% and 11.2%.[78]

COMPARATIVE STUDIES

FDG-PET does not provide information about the specific pathology of AD, unlike the data provided by PIB or FDDNP-PET. Still, numerous reports demonstrate that FDG-PET shows a typical AD functional pattern that can also be distinguished in patients with MCI, particularly those with aMCI; besides, this pattern has been able to predict the conversion from NL to MCI[31,37] and from MCI to AD, with high accuracy rates.[32,37,38,48,49,51] PIB binding shows a more

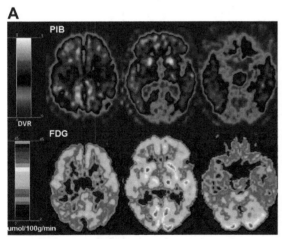 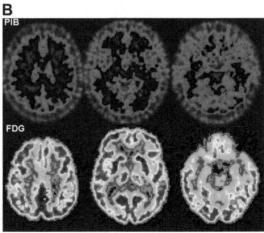

Fig. 1. PIB and FDG-PET scans from 2 representative subjects. (*A*) A 71-year-old male AD subject, GDS 5, MMSE 19. (*B*) A 65-year-old male NL subject, GDS 1, MMSE 29. (*Top row*) PIB-PET images; (*bottom row*) coregistered FDG-PET images. PET scans are displayed in the axial plane, from the top to the bottom of the brain, at the level of the centrum semiovale (*left*), basal ganglia (*center*), and medial temporal lobe (*right*). GDS, global deterioration scale; MMSE, Mini-Mental State Examination. (*Reproduced from* Li Y, Rinne JO, Mosconi L, et al. Regional analysis of FDG and PIB-PET images in normal aging, mild cognitive impairment, and Alzheimer's disease. Eur J Nucl Med Mol Imaging 2008;35(12):2169–81; with permission.)

extensive retention in the neocortex and striatum.[95] As with FDG-PET studies, PIB positivity in patients with MCI has predicted the conversion to probable AD.[97,98] Only a few studies have compared different radioligands and their properties in the same patients with MCI.

Comparisons Between PIB and FDG-PET

Only 2 ROI analysis studies have directly compared the diagnostic separation of defined clinical categories between PIB and FDG-PET (**Fig. 1**, **Table 4**).[90,98] Both showed similar accuracy in separating cognitively impaired subjects into the defined clinical categories. In Lowe and colleagues'[98] study on 20 NL, 23 MCI (17 aMCI, 6 nonamnestic), and 13 AD subjects, PIB and FDG-PET showed similar accuracy in characterizing control, AD, and MCI groups, whereas in Li and colleagues'[90] study on 7 NL, 13 MCI, and 17 AD patients, FDG-PET showed a better performance in the classification of NL, MCI, and AD subjects with the Hip as the most significant group discriminator. Various differences between both studies may explain the dissimilar results, including the use of a fully quantitative FDG metabolic glucose rate calculation and a small group of normal elderly by Li and colleagues[90] and the use of 2 groups of patients with MCI by Lowe and colleagues.[98] In Li and colleagues'[90] study, the combination of the 2 PET techniques improved the diagnostic accuracy of MCI to 90%.

Comparisons Between PIB and FDDNP-PET

Only 2 studies have directly compared global and regional uptake of PIB and FDDNP in the same subjects in samples of NL versus MCI or AD[92] and NL versus AD.[99] In Tolboom and colleagues'[92] study on 13 NL controls and 14 AD and 11 aMCI patients, PIB binding was found to be better at discriminating among NL, aMCI, and AD groups, whereas FDDNP uptake was higher only in patients with AD compared with subjects with MCI and NL (**Fig. 2**). Shin and colleagues[99] reported in 10 patients with AD and 10 controls that medial temporal cortex (Hip, amygdala, and parahippocampal gyrus) PIB binding was found to be negligible in patients with AD, whereas FDDNP binding was elevated, with significant uptake of both tracers in the other AD-vulnerable neocortical areas. This is seen as a proof of FDDNP distinctive binding, as the MTL displays extensive NFT and few Aβ plaques.

Table 4
Comparative studies of FGD and PIB-PET

References	Subjects	PIB group Differences (P<.05)	FDG group Differences (P<.05)	Method	Conclusions
Li et al,[90] 2008	7 NL, 13 MCI, and 17 AD	NL vs AD MCI vs AD	NL vs AD NL vs MCI MCI vs AD	ROI	In the classification of NL, AD, and MCI, FDG showed slightly better separation of subjects compared with PIB. Combining the 2 modalities improves the diagnostic accuracy for MCI. The diagnostically most useful PIB region was the middle frontal gyrus, and the most useful CMRglc reductions were found in the hippocampus
Lowe et al,[98] 2009	20 normal elderly, 17 aMCI, 6 naMCI, and 13 AD subjects	NL vs AD naMCI vs aMCI, naMCI vs ADaMCI vs AD	NL vs AD naMCI vs AD aMCI vs AD	ROI	In the classification of NL, aMCI, naMCI, and AD, PIB showed slightly better separation of subjects between aMCI and naMCI compared with FDG

Abbreviation: ROI: region of interest analysis.

A

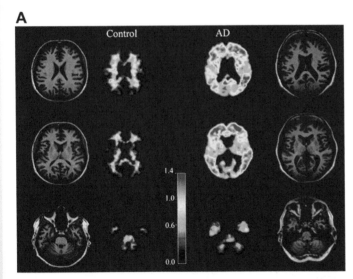

B

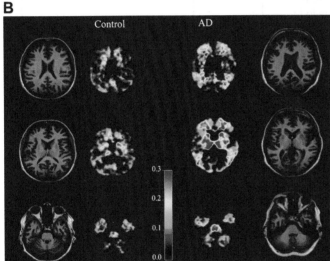

Fig. 2. Examples of parametric ^{11}C-PIB (*A*) and ^{18}F-FDDNP (*B*) parametric images of bonding potential (BP$_{ND}$) in healthy control and AD patient. ^{11}C-PIB and ^{18}F-FDDNP scans were acquired in same subjects. In each panel, control is on the left and the patient with AD is on the right. High level of ^{18}F-FDDNP binding in subcortical structures suggests nonspecific binding. (*Reproduced from* Tolboom N, Yaqub M, van der Flier WM, et al. Detection of Alzheimer pathology in vivo using both 11C-PIB and 18F-FDDNP PET. J Nucl Med 2009;50(2):191–7; with permission.)

LIMITATIONS
Visual Reading

One limitation to the use of PET in the clinical practice is the reliance on qualitative interpretation of the images by visual reading. Studies have shown that more consistent and accurate data are obtained using quantitative evaluations of FDG-PET scans. This is especially the case if used to determine the progression of the CMRglc decrease. However, in clinical practice, arterial blood sampling during the examination is rarely performed, making impossible the quantitative evaluation of FDG-PET scans. FDG and amyloid PET measures often lack clearly defined cutoffs to distinguish between normal and pathologic findings. Thus, scans are interpreted by visual analysis, which depends on the experience and training of the observer and has high interobserver variability. The percentage of change between the NL and AD groups is much greater for PIB than for FDG or FDDNP tracers in the different brain ROIs where this separation is expected; so a better visual separation into PIB positive and negative binding is assumed for this tracer, with a higher interobserver agreement and with an accuracy exceeding 90%, far greater than those shown with FDG-PET.[100,101] Identification of increased uptake in individual cases may also prove to be difficult with FDDNP,[92,93] suggesting that the accuracy of FDDNP as a differential diagnostic tool for the detection of Alzheimer pathology in individual subjects might be difficult. Moreover, even with PIB, the identification of a mildly increased gray matter uptake could be hard, because the nonspecific white matter uptake could overwhelm it. To address some of these difficulties, Mosconi

Table 5
PET studies and differential diagnosis against AD

Diagnosis	FDG	PIB	References
FTLD	Anterior-predominant hypometabolism (prefrontal and anteriotemporal cortex)	20%–33% of the FTLD patients are PIB+	101,103–106
LBD	Occipital hypometabolism, in addition to TP	AD pattern: increased uptake in the frontal, PCC temporoparietal, occipital cortices and in the striatum	102,107–110
VD	Focal subcortical and cortical hypometabolism	No studies	111
aMCI	Hypometabolism in PCC, parietotemporal cortices and MTL	Increased biding in frontal, anterior cingulate, precuneus, and lateral temporoparietal cortices	33,36–38,40,88
Non-aMCI	Variable, ranging from isolated Hip CMRglc reductions to metabolic patterns consistent with different types of dementia, such as FTLD and LBD	Similar distribution of PIB binding to that of the aMCI patients	31,32,41,45,88
Depression	Frontal hypometabolism	No studies	112

Abbreviation: TP, temporoparietal.

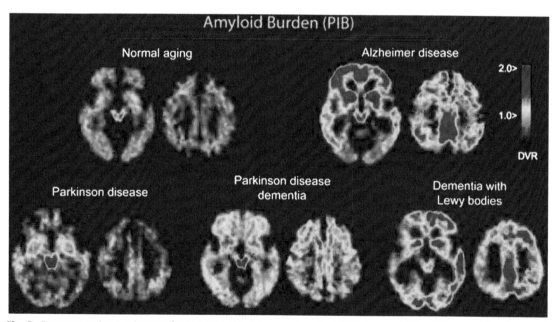

Fig. 3. Representative PIB images from a 75-year-old normal control (NC) (*upper left*), a 79-year-old patient with Alzheimer disease (AD) (MMSE score 25; *upper right*), a 65-year-old patient with Parkinson disease (PD) (MMSE score 27; *lower left*), a 69-year-old patient with PD dementia (PDD) (MMSE score 25; *lower middle*), and a 71-year-old patient with dementia with Lewy bodies (DLB) (MMSE score 8; *lower right*) are displayed. Note that Pittsburgh compound-B retention is qualitatively increased in AD, PDD, and DLB compared with NC and PD. Note also the variation in the regional distribution of amyloid across the AD, PDD, and DLB images. DVR, distribution volume ratio. (*Reproduced from* Gomperts SN, Rentz DM, Moran E, et al. Imaging amyloid deposition in Lewy body diseases. Neurology 2008;71(12):903–10; with permission.)

and colleagues[44] have developed and validated a FDG-PET visual rating scale for MTL hypometabolism, which is useful for the examination of patients at the MCI stage and as accurate as the quantitative evaluations of scans.

Tracers' Characteristics

The use of PIB in clinical practice could be limited by the fact that this tracer is labeled with ^{11}C; because of its short physical half-life (about 20 minutes), its use is restricted only to hospitals with an on-site cyclotron. Instead, tracers labeled with [18]F (half-life of about 2 hours), such as FDDNP or other amyloid tracers in development and of course FDG, are much more suitable for the use in routine clinical practice. Indeed, ^{18}F-labeled radiotracers can be easily shipped from a center with a cyclotron to the nearby nuclear medicine departments, thus making these tracers available for all PET centers. Besides, several ^{18}F-labeled Aβ tracers have recently been developed and are currently under clinical evaluation.

Diagnostic Specificity

Another limitation of PET tracers is the lack of diagnostic specificity. Several FDG-PET studies have aimed to identify specific patterns for different neurodegenerative diseases. Patients with LBD show a more prominent hypometabolism in the occipital cortices compared with those with AD, whereas patients with FTLD show more prominent hypometabolism in the frontal or temporal cortices.[102,103] However, patients with LBD and FTLD often show a pattern of cortical deficits similar to that of patients with AD (FDG-PET findings in DLB, FTLD, and other dementias are shown in **Table 5**). Therefore, the presence of cortical abnormalities discriminates AD from LBD and FTLD, with a high sensitivity (>90%), although with a lower specificity (71% and 65%, respectively).[41] PIB is a specific marker for pathologic brain amyloid structures,[102] but lacks diagnostic specificity, as amyloid load is common in the aging population and can be detected in cerebral amyloid angiopathy.[82,87,103] Most studies report high sensitivity, with specificity determined by the age of the patient, ranging from 73% to 96%.[99] PIB retention has been found in the AD range in 58% of patients with aMCI and 43% of those with nonamnestic MCI,[88] and increases in cortical PIB have been reported in 40% to 85% of patients with LBD,[84,107,108,113] 17% to 33% with Parkinson disease dementia (PDD),[107,114] and 20% to 25% with FTLD.[101,108,114] These findings somehow reproduce neuropathologic findings, as it can be estimated that about one-

fourth of the patients with Lewy body disease suffer also from cortical Aβ burden, with the highest proportion in LBD subjects, followed by PDD subjects (**Fig. 3**),[114,115] and comorbid AD and FTLD pathology, while relatively uncommon, can be seen on autopsy. Conversely, about 15% to 20% of demented patients with enough cortical Aβ plaques and NFT to meet neuropathologic criteria for AD also have cortical and subcortical Lewy bodies that are previously thought to be pathognomonic for Parkinson disease; furthermore, some patients with underlying AD pathology can mimic an FTLD clinical phenotype or show any other atypical presentations.[16]

SUMMARY

Patients with early cognitive symptoms constitute a biologically heterogeneous population that needs to be better defined and characterized. The postmortem neuropathologic definitive diagnosis of AD also has uncertainties because of the phenotypic heterogeneity of the disease; the coexistence with other pathologies, such as LBD or VD[116]; and the overlap of AD lesions with those observed in normal aging and MCI in the absence of a normative aging morphology. PET imaging findings help to disentangle both sources of variability. As reviewed in this article, there is growing evidence that FDG and PIB-PET accurately distinguish AD from normal aging, precede cognitive decline, predict conversion to dementia, and are increasingly consistent with the known histology of the disease.[23,88,109]

The prognostic value of a PIB positive or negative scan result may have different clinical connotations in patients with MCI. PIB positive MCI patients have a high risk of developing AD, whereas PIB negative MCI patients can revert to "cognitively normal" or have prodromal dementias other than AD. Newly defined PET groups, such as PIB negative aMCI or PIB positive nonamnestic MCI, enrich the construct and the current clinical categorical classification of MCI and serve as a promising approach to better understand MCI as a diagnostic entity and as a risk factor for future cognitive decline. These encouraging results should be more thoroughly studied in terms of clinical relevance, stability, and specific outcomes because the studies are still modest in several patients and there is some variability in terms of diagnostic groups, cutoffs for the designation of amyloid-positivity, and duration of the clinical follow-ups.

Currently, the clinical diagnosis of AD in predementia stages is symptom based, without any accepted confirmatory laboratory protocols available. Neuroimaging has the potential to independently and accurately confirm clinical impressions, although there remains a great need to increase the diagnostic accuracy and to study the specificity of PET tracers against neuro-pathology. Further longitudinal observation, coupled with different tracers (eg, combination of FDG with amyloid ligands) may be an effective strategy in the identification of these early stages. These subjects would be the ideal therapeutic target for prevention strategies or any disease-modifying drug that may potentially abort or delay the onset of the cognitive decline.

REFERENCES

1. Alzheimer's Association. 2009 Alzheimer's disease facts and figures. Alzheimer's Dement 2009;5(3): 234–70.
2. Braak H, Braak E. Neuropathological stageing of Alzheimer-related changes. Acta Neuropathol 1991;82:239–59.
3. Morris JC, Storandt M, Miller JP, et al. Mild cognitive impairment represents early stage Alzheimer's disease. Arch Neurol 2001;58:397–405.
4. Thal DR, Capetillo-Zarate E, Del Tredici K, et al. The development of amyloid beta protein deposits in the aged brain. Sci Aging Knowledge Environ 2006;8(6):1–7.
5. Graham JE, Rockwood K, Beattie BL, et al. Prevalence and severity of cognitive impairment with and without dementia in an elderly population. Lancet 1997;349(9068):1793–6.
6. Dubois B. 'Prodromal Alzheimer's disease': a more useful concept than mild cognitive impairment? Curr Opin Neurol 2000;13(4):367–9.
7. Morris JC. The Clinical Dementia Rating (CDR): current version and scoring rules. Neurology 1993;43:2412–4.
8. Reisberg B, Ferris SH, Kluger A, et al. Mild cognitive impairment (MCI): a historical perspective. Int Psychogeriatr 2008;20(1):18–31.
9. Ritchie K, Touchon J. Mild cognitive impairment: conceptual basis and current nosological status. Lancet 2000;355(9199):225–8.
10. Mariani E, Monastero R, Mecocci P. Mild cognitive impairment: a systematic review. J Alzheimers Dis 2007;12(1):23–35.
11. Winblad B, Palmer K, Kivipelto M, et al. Mild cognitive impairment–beyond controversies, towards a consensus: report of the International Working Group on Mild Cognitive Impairment. J Intern Med 2004;256(3):240–6.
12. Petersen RC, Smith GE, Waring SC, et al. Mild cognitive impairment: clinical characterization and outcomes. Arch Neurol 1999;56(3):303–8.
13. Ganguli M, Dodge HH, Shen C, et al. Mild cognitive impairment, amnestic type: an epidemiologic study. Neurology 2004;63(1):115–21.
14. Boyle PA, Wilson RS, Aggarwal NT, et al. Mild cognitive impairment: risk of Alzheimer disease and rate of cognitive decline. Neurology 2006; 67(3):441–5.
15. Petersen RC, Doody R, Kurz A, et al. Current concepts in mild cognitive impairment. Arch Neurol 2001;58:1985–92.
16. Galton CJ, Patterson K, Xuereb JH, et al. Atypical and typical presentations of Alzheimer's disease: a clinical, neuropsychological, neuroimaging and pathological study of 13 cases. Brain 2000; 123(3):484–98.
17. Busse A, Hensel A, Guhne U, et al. Mild cognitive impairment: long-term course of four clinical subtypes. Neurology 2006;67:2176–85.
18. Haroutunian V, Hoffman LB, Beeri MS, et al. Is there a neuropathology difference between mild cognitive impairment and dementia? Dialogues Clin Neurosci 2009;11(2):171–9.
19. Petersen RC, Parisi JE, Dickson DW, et al. Neuro-pathologic features of amnestic mild cognitive impairment. Arch Neurol 2006;63(5):665–72.
20. Reisberg B, Prichep L, Mosconi L, et al. The pre-mild cognitive impairment, subjective cognitive impairment stage of Alzheimer's disease. Alzheimers Dement 2008;4(1 Suppl 1):S98–108.
21. Whitehouse PJ. Mild cognitive impairment–a confused concept? Nat Clin Pract Neurol 2007; 3(2):62–3.
22. Mosconi L. Brain glucose metabolism in the early and specific diagnosis of Alzheimer's disease. FDG-PET studies in MCI and AD. Eur J Nucl Med Mol Imaging 2005;32(4):486–510.
23. Silverman DH, Small GW, Chang CY, et al. Positron emission tomography in evaluation of dementia: regional brain metabolism and long-term outcome. JAMA 2001;286(17):2120–7.
24. Mosconi L, Mistur R, Switalski R, et al. FDG-PET changes in brain glucose metabolism from normal cognition to pathologically verified Alzheimer's disease. Eur J Nucl Med Mol Imaging 2009;36(5): 811–22.
25. Ikonomovic MD, Klunk WE, Abrahamson EE, et al. Post-mortem correlates of in vivo PiB-PET amyloid imaging in a typical case of Alzheimer's disease. Brain 2008;131(Pt 6):1630–45.
26. De Leon MJ, Ferris SH, George AE, et al. Computed tomography evaluations of brain-behavior relationships in senile dementia of the Alzheimer's type. Neurobiol Aging 1980;1(1): 69–79.
27. Sokoloff L. Relation between physiological functions and energy metabolism in the central nervous system. J Neurochem 1977;29:13–26.

28. Attwell D, Iadecola C. The neural basis of functional brain imaging signals. Trends Neurosci 2002; 25(12):621–5.

29. Gomez-Isla T, Price JL, McKeel DW Jr, et al. Profound loss of layer II entorhinal cortex neurons occurs in very mild Alzheimer's disease. J Neurosci 1996;16:4491–500.

30. Herholz K. PET studies in dementia. Ann Nucl Med 2003;17(2):79–89.

31. de Leon MJ, Convit A, Wolf OT, et al. Prediction of cognitive decline in normal elderly subjects with 2-[18F]fluoro-2-deoxy-D-glucose/positron-emission tomography (FDG/PET). Proc Natl Acad Sci U S A 2001;98:10966–71.

32. De Santi S, de Leon MJ, Rusinek H, et al. Hippocampal formation glucose metabolism and volume losses in MCI and AD. Neurobiol Aging 2001;22: 529–39.

33. Minoshima S, Giordani B, Berent S, et al. Metabolic reduction in the posterior cingulate cortex in very early Alzheimer's disease. Ann Neurol 1997;42(1): 85–94.

34. Friedland RP, Brun A, Budinger TF. Pathological and positron emission tomographic correlations in Alzheimer's disease. Lancet 1985;26:228.

35. Pardo JV, Lee JT, Sheikh SA, et al. Where the brain grows old: decline in anterior cingulate and medial prefrontal function with normal aging. Neuroimage 2007;35(3):1231–7.

36. Nestor PJ, Scheltens P, Hodges JR, et al. Advances in the early detection of Alzheimer's disease. Nat Med 2004;10(Suppl):S34–41.

37. Chételat G, Desgranges B, de la Sayette V, et al. Mild cognitive impairment: can FDG-PET predict who is to rapidly convert to Alzheimer's disease? Neurology 2003;60(8):1374–7.

38. Drzezga A, Lautenschlager N, Siebner H, et al. Cerebral metabolic changes accompanying conversion of mild cognitive impairment into Alzheimer's disease: a PET follow-up study. Eur J Nucl Med Mol Imaging 2003;30:1104–13.

39. Mosconi L, Perani D, Sorbi S, et al. MCI conversion to dementia and the APOE genotype: a prediction study with FDG-PET. Neurology 2004;63:2332–40.

40. Langbaum JB, Chen K, Lee W, et al. Categorical and correlational analyses of baseline fluorodeoxyglucose positron emission tomography images from the Alzheimer's Disease Neuroimaging Initiative (ADNI). Neuroimage 2009;45:1107–16.

41. Mosconi L, Tsui WH, Herholz K, et al. Multicenter standardized 18F-FDG PET diagnosis of mild cognitive impairment, Alzheimer's disease, and other dementias. J Nucl Med 2008;49(3):390–8.

42. Alexopoulos P, Grimmer T, Perneczky R, et al. Progression to dementia in clinical subtypes of mild cognitive impairment. Progression to dementia in clinical subtypes of mild cognitive impairment. Dement Geriatr Cogn Disord 2006; 22(1):27–34.

43. Berent S, Giordani B, Foster N, et al. Neuropsychological function and cerebral glucose utilization in isolated memory impairment and Alzheimer's disease. J Psychiatr Res 1999;33(1):7–16.

44. Mosconi L, De Santi S, Li Y, et al. Visual rating of medial temporal lobe metabolism in mild cognitive impairment and Alzheimer's disease using FDG-PET. Eur J Nucl Med Mol Imaging 2006; 33:210–21.

45. Reed BR, Jagust WJ, Seab JP, et al. Memory and regional cerebral blood flow in mildly symptomatic Alzheimer's disease. Neurology 1989;39: 1537–9.

46. Jagust W, Gitcho A, Sun F, et al. Brain imaging evidence of preclinical Alzheimer's disease in normal aging. Ann Neurol 2006;59(4):673–81.

47. Mosconi L, De Santi S, Li J, et al. Hippocampal hypometabolism predicts cognitive decline from normal aging. Neurobiol Aging 2008;29(5):676–92.

48. Herholz K, Nordberg A, Salmon E, et al. Impairment of neocortical metabolism predicts progression in Alzheimer's disease. Dement Geriatr Cogn Disord 1999;10:494–504.

49. Arnáiz E, Jelic V, Almkvist O, et al. Impaired cerebral glucose metabolism and cognitive functioning predict deterioration in mild cognitive impairment. Neuroreport 2001;12(4):851–5.

50. Silverman DH, Truong CT, Kim SK, et al. Prognostic value of regional cerebral metabolism in patients undergoing dementia evaluation: comparison to a quantifying parameter of subsequent cognitive performance and to prognostic assessment without PET. Mol Genet Metab 2003;80:350–5.

51. Anchisi D, Borroni B, Franceschi M, et al. Heterogeneity of brain glucose metabolism in mild cognitive impairment and clinical progression to Alzheimer disease. Arch Neurol 2005;62:1728–33.

52. Drzezga A, Grimmer T, Riemenschneider M, et al. Prediction of individual clinical outcome in MCI by means of genetic assessment and (18)F-FDG PET. J Nucl Med 2005;46(10):1625–32.

53. Fouquet M, Desgranges B, Landeau B, et al. Longitudinal brain metabolic changes from amnestic mild cognitive impairment to Alzheimer's disease. Brain 2009;132:2058–67.

54. Yuan Y, Gu ZX, Wei WS. Fluorodeoxyglucose-positron-emission tomography, single-photon emission tomography, and structural MR imaging for prediction of rapid conversion to Alzheimer disease in patients with mild cognitive impairment: a meta-analysis. AJNR Am J Neuroradiol 2009;30:404–10.

55. Corder EH, Saunders AM, Strittmatter WJ, et al. Gene dose of apolipoprotein E type 4 allele and

the risk of Alzheimer's disease in late onset families. Science 1993;261(5123):921–3.

56. Farrer LA, Cupples LA, Haines JL, et al. Effects of age, sex, and ethnicity on the association between apolipoprotein E genotype and Alzheimer disease. JAMA 1997;278(16):1349–56.

57. Laws SM, Hone E, Gandy S, et al. Expanding the association between the APOE gene and the risk of Alzheimer's disease: possible roles for APOE promoter polymorphisms and alterations in APOE transcription. J Neurochem 2003;84:1215–36.

58. Mosconi L, De Santi S, Brys M, et al. Hypometabolism and altered CSF markers in normal ApoE E4 carriers with subjective memory complaints. Biol Psychiatry 2008;63(6):609–18.

59. Reiman EM, Caselli RJ, Yun LS, et al. Preclinical evidence of Alzheimer's disease in persons homozygous for the E4 allele for apolipoprotein E. N Engl J Med 1996;334:752–8.

60. Reiman EM, Caselli RJ, Chen K, et al. Declining brain activity in cognitively normal apolipoprotein E epsilon 4 heterozygotes: a foundation for using positron emission tomography to efficiently test treatments to prevent Alzheimer's disease. Proc Natl Acad Sci U S A 2001;98:3334–9.

61. Reiman EM, Chen K, Alexander GE, et al. Functional brain abnormalities in young adults at genetic risk for late-onset Alzheimer's dementia. Proc Natl Acad Sci U S A 2004;101:284–9.

62. Reiman EM, Uecker A, Caselli RJ, et al. Hippocampal volumes in cognitively normal persons at genetic risk for Alzheimer's disease. Ann Neurol 1998;44:288–91.

63. Small GW, Mazziotta JC, Collins MT, et al. Apolipoprotein E type 4 allele and cerebral glucose metabolism in relatives at risk for familial Alzheimer disease. JAMA 1995;273:942–7.

64. Caselli RJ, Reiman EM, Locke DE, et al. Cognitive domain decline in healthy apolipoprotein E epsilon4 homozygotes before the diagnosis of mild cognitive impairment. Arch Neurol 2007;64: 1306–11.

65. Reiman EM, Chen K, Alexander GE, et al. Correlations between apolipoprotein E epsilon4 gene dose and brain-imaging measurements of regional hypometabolism. Proc Natl Acad Sci U S A 2005; 102(23):8299–302.

66. Gottesman II, Gould TD. The endophenotype concept in psychiatry: etymology and strategic intentions. Am J Psychiatry 2003;160(4):636–45.

67. Farrer LA, Cupples LA, Haines JL, et al. Effects of age, sex, and ethnicity on the association between apolipoprotein E genotype and Alzheimer disease. A meta-analysis. APOE and Alzheimer Disease Meta Analysis Consortium. JAMA 1997;278(16):1349–56.

68. Cupples LA, Farrer LA, Sadovnik AD, et al. Estimating risk curves for first-degree relatives of

patients with Alzheimer's disease: the REVEAL study. Genet Med 2004;6(4):192–6.

69. Green RC, Cupples LA, Go R, et al. MIRAGE Study Group. Risk of dementia among white and African American relatives of patients with Alzheimer disease. JAMA 2002;287(3):329–36.

70. Silverman JM, Ciresi G, Smith CJ, et al. Variability of familial risk of Alzheimer disease across the late life span. Arch Gen Psychiatry 2005;62(5): 565–73.

71. Edland SD, Silverman JM, Peskind ER, et al. Increased risk of dementia in mothers of Alzheimer's disease cases: evidence for maternal inheritance. Neurology 1996;47:254–6.

72. Ehrenkrantz D, Silverman JM, Smith CJ, et al. Genetic epidemiological study of maternal and paternal transmission of Alzheimer's disease. Am J Med Genet 1999;88:378–82.

73. Mosconi L, Brys M, Switalski R, et al. Maternal family history of Alzheimer's disease predisposes to reduced brain glucose metabolism. Proc Natl Acad Sci U S A 2007;104:19067–72.

74. Mosconi L, Mistur R, Switalski R, et al. Declining brain glucose metabolism in normal individuals with a maternal history of Alzheimer disease. Neurology 2009;72:513–20.

75. Swerdlow RH. PET sheds light on Alzheimer's disease genetic risk. Proc Natl Acad Sci U S A 2007;104:18881–2.

76. Klunk WE, Engler H, Nordberg A, et al. Imaging brain amyloid in Alzheimer's disease with Pittsburgh Compound-B. Ann Neurol 2004;55:306–19.

77. Agdeppa ED, Kepe V, Liu J, et al. Binding characteristics of radiofluorinated 6-dialkylamino-2-naphthylethylidene derivatives as positron emission tomography imaging probes for beta-amyloid plaques in Alzheimer's disease. J Neurosci 2001;21: 1–5.

78. Small GW, Kepe V, Ercoli LM, et al. PET of brain amyloid and tau in mild cognitive impairment. N Engl J Med 2006;355:2652–63.

79. Verhoeff NP, Wilson AA, Takeshita S, et al. In-vivo imaging of Alzheimer disease beta-amyloid with [11C]SB-13 PET. Am J Geriatr Psychiatry 2004; 12:584–95.

80. Kudo Y, Okamura N, Forumoto S, et al. 2-(2-[2-Dimethylaminothiazol-5-yl] ethenyl)-6-(2-[fluoro]ethoxy)benzoxazole: a novel PET agent for in vivo detection of dense amyloid plaques in Alzheimer's disease patients. J Nucl Med 2007;49: 554–61.

81. Rowe CC, Ackerman U, Browne W, et al. Imaging of amyloid beta in Alzheimer's disease with (18)F-BAY94-9172, a novel PET tracer: proof of mechanism. Lancet Neurol 2008;7:129–35.

82. Mintun MAM, LaRossa GN, Sheline YIM, et al. [11C]PIB in a nondemented population: potential

antecedent marker of Alzheimer disease. Neurology 2006;67:446–52.

83. Pike KE, Savage G, Villemagne V, et al. Beta-amyloid imaging and memory in non-demented individuals: evidence for preclinical Alzheimer's disease. Brain 2007;130:2837–44.

84. Rowe CC, Ng S, Ackermann U, et al. Imaging beta-amyloid burden in aging and dementia. Neurology 2007;68:1718–25.

85. Kemppainen N, Aalto S, Wilson I, et al. Voxel-based analysis of PET amyloid ligand [11C]PIB uptake in Alzheimer disease. Neurology 2006;67:1575–80.

86. Forsberg A, Engler H, Almkvist O, et al. PET imaging of amyloid deposition in patients with mild cognitive impairment. Neurobiol Aging 2008; 29(10):1456–65.

87. Aizenstein HJ, Nebes RD, Saxton JA, et al. Frequent amyloid deposition without significant cognitive impairment among the elderly. Arch Neurol 2008;65(11):1509–17.

88. Wolk DA, Price JC, Saxton JA, et al. Amyloid imaging in mild cognitive impairment subtypes. Ann Neurol 2009;65:557–68.

89. Grimmer T, Riemenschneider M, Förstl H. Beta amyloid in Alzheimer's disease: increased deposition in brain is reflected in reduced concentration in cerebrospinal fluid. Biol Psychiatry 2009; 65(11):927–34.

90. Li Y, Rinne JO, Mosconi L, et al. Regional analysis of FDG and PIB-PET images in normal aging, mild cognitive impairment, and Alzheimer's disease. Eur J Nucl Med Mol Imaging 2008;35: 2169–81.

91. Shoghi-Jadid K, Small D, Agdeppa ED, et al. Localization of neurofibrillary tangles and beta-amyloid plaques in the brain of living patients with Alzheimer disease. Am J Geriatr Psychiatry 2002;10:24–35.

92. Tolboom N, Yaqub M, van der Flier WM. Detection of Alzheimer pathology in vivo using both 11C-PIB and 18F-FDDNP PET. J Nucl Med 2009;50(2): 191–7.

93. de Leon MJ, Mosconi L, Logan J. Seeing what Alzheimer saw. Nat Med 2007;13:129–31.

94. Engler H, Forsberg A, Almkvist O, et al. Two-year follow-up of amyloid deposition in patients with Alzheimer's disease. Brain 2006;129(Pt 11):2856–66.

95. Kemppainen NM, Aalto S, Wilson IA, et al. PET amyloid ligand [11C]PIB uptake is increased in mild cognitive impairment. Neurology 2007; 68(19):1603–6.

96. Koivunen J, Pirttilä T, Kemppainen N, et al. PET amyloid ligand [11C]PIB uptake and cerebrospinal fluid beta-amyloid in mild cognitive impairment. Dement Geriatr Cogn Disord 2008;26(4): 378–83.

97. Okello A, Koivunen J, Edison P, et al. Conversion of amyloid positive and negative MCI to AD over 3 years. An 11C-PIB PET study. Neurology 2009; 73(10):754–60.

98. Lowe VJ, Kemp BJ, Jack CR, et al. Comparison of 18F-FDG and PiB PET in cognitive impairment. J Nucl Med 2009;50:878–86.

99. Shin J, Lee SY, Kim SH. Multitracer PET imaging of amyloid plaques and neurofibrillary tangles in Alzheimer's disease. Neuroimage 2008;43(2): 236–44.

100. Ng S, Villemagne VL, Berlangieri S, et al. Visual assessment versus quantitative assessment of 11C-PIB PET and 18F-FDG PET for detection of Alzheimer's disease. J Nucl Med 2007;48(4): 547–52.

101. Rabinovici GD, Furst AJ, O'Neil JP, et al. 11C-PIB PET imaging in Alzheimer disease and frontotemporal lobar degeneration. Neurology 2007;68(15): 1205–12.

102. Minoshima S, Foster NL, Sima AA, et al. Alzheimer's disease versus dementia with Lewy bodies: cerebral metabolic distinction with autopsy confirmation. Ann Neurol 2001;50:358–65.

103. Diehl-Schmid J, Grimmer T, Drzezga A, et al. Decline of cerebral glucose metabolism in frontotemporal dementia: a longitudinal 18F-FDG-PET-study. Neurobiol Aging 2007;28:42–50.

104. Engler H, Santillo AF, Wang SX, et al. In vivo amyloid imaging with PET in frontotemporal dementia. Eur J Nucl Med Mol Imaging 2008; 35(1):100–6.

105. Drzezga A, Grimmer T, Henriksen G, et al. Imaging of amyloid plaques and cerebral glucose metabolism in semantic dementia and Alzheimer's disease. Neuroimage 2008;39(2):619–33.

106. Ishii K, Sakamoto S, Sasaki M, et al. Cerebral glucose metabolism in patients with frontotemporal dementia. J Nucl Med 1998;39:1875–8.

107. Edison P, Rowe CC, Rinne JO, et al. Amyloid load in Parkinson's disease dementia and Lewy Body dementia measured with [11C]PIB PET. J Neurol Neurosurg Psychiatr 2008;79:1331–8.

108. Gomperts SN, Rentz DM, Moran E, et al. Imaging amyloid deposition in Lewy body diseases. Neurology 2008;71(12):903–10.

109. Mosconi L, Brys M, Glodzik-Sobanska L, et al. Early detection of Alzheimer's disease using neuroimaging. Exp Gerontol 2007;42(1–2):129–38.

110. Albin RL, Minoshima S, D'Amato CJ, et al. Fluorodeoxyglucose positron emission tomography in diffuse Lewy body disease. Neurology 1996;47: 462–6.

111. Szelies B, Mielke R, Herholz K, et al. Quantitative topographical EEG compared to FDG PET for classification of vascular and degenerative dementia.

Electroencephalogr Clin Neurophysiol 1994;91:131–9.

112. Guze BH, Baxter LR Jr, Schwartz JM, et al. Changes in glucose metabolism in dementia of the Alzheimer type compared with depression: a preliminary report. Psychiatry Res 1991;40:195–202.

113. Lockhart A, Lamb JR, Osredkar T, et al. PIB is a non-specific imaging marker of amyloid-beta (Abeta) peptide-related cerebral amyloidosis. Brain 2007;130(Pt 10):2607–15.

114. Maetzler W, Liepelt I, Reimold M, et al. Cortical PIB binding in Lewy body disease is associated with Alzheimer-like characteristics. Neurobiol Dis 2009; 34(1):107–12.

115. Hughes AJ, Daniel SE, Blankson S, et al. A clinico-pathologic study of 100 cases of Parkinson's disease. Arch Neurol 1993;50:140–8.

116. Jellinger KA, Bancher C. Neuropathology of Alzheimer's disease: a critical update. J Neural Transm Suppl 1998;54:77–95.

Amyloid PET Ligands for Dementia

Victor L. Villemagne, MD[a,b,c,]*, Christopher C. Rowe, MD[a,c]

KEYWORDS
- Alzheimer's disease • Aβ • Brain imaging
- Positron emission tomography

ALZHEIMER'S DISEASE AND OTHER DEMENTIAS

Alzheimer's disease (AD), the most common cause of dementia in the elderly, is an irreversible, progressive neurodegenerative disorder clinically characterized by memory loss as well as cognitive and functional decline that leads invariably to death, usually within 7 to 10 years after diagnosis.[1] The disease not only has devastating effects on the sufferers and their caregivers, but also has a tremendous socioeconomic impact on families and the health system.[2–4] The progressive nature of neurodegeneration suggests an age-dependent process that ultimately leads to synaptic failure and neuronal damage in cortical areas of the brain critical for memory and higher mental functions.[5,6] The increasing age of the population in developed countries suggests that, if unchecked, these disorders will become increasingly prevalent.

In the absence of specific biologic markers, direct pathologic examination of brain tissue still is the only definitive method for establishing a diagnosis of AD.[6,7] The typical macroscopic picture is gross cortical atrophy while microscopically, there is widespread cellular degeneration and diffuse synaptic and neuronal loss, accompanied by reactive gliosis and the presence of the pathologic hallmarks of the disease: intracellular neurofibrillary tangles (NFT) and extracellular amyloid plaques.[6–8]

Whereas NFT are intraneuronal bundles of paired helical filaments mainly composed of the aggregates of an abnormally phosphorylated form of tau protein,[9,10] neuritic plaques consist of dense extracellular aggregates of β-amyloid (Aβ),[11] surrounded by reactive gliosis and dystrophic neurites. Aβ is a 4-kDa 39- to 43-amino acid metalloprotein derived from the proteolytic cleavage of the amyloid precursor protein (APP), by β- and γ-secretases.[12] To date, all available evidence strongly supports the notion that an imbalance between the production and removal of Aβ leading to its progressive accumulation is central to the pathogenesis of AD.[13]

Postmortem studies have shown that the distribution and density of both diffuse (amorphous β deposits and not associated with dystrophic neurites and glial reaction) and neuritic β plaques have not been consistently shown to correlate with the degree of cognitive impairment in AD.[14,15] In contrast, the best physiologic correlation has been observed with NFT and soluble levels of Aβ.[16–21] These soluble forms of Aβ, in equilibrium with the insoluble Aβ in plaques, are potentially neurotoxic through several possible mechanisms, including: oxidative stress, excitotoxicity, energy depletion, toxic oxidative interaction with various metal species, inflammatory response, and apoptosis.[13] Nevertheless, the exact toxic mechanism by which Aβ effects synaptic loss and neuronal death is still controversial.[1,22,23]

At present, the clinical diagnosis of AD is based on progressive impairment of memory, decline in at least one other cognitive domain affecting the

This work was supported in part by grant 509166 of the National Health and Medical Research Council of Australia, and the Austin Hospital Medical Research Foundation, and Neurosciences Victoria.
[a] Department of Nuclear Medicine and Centre for PET, Austin Health, 145 Studley Road, Heidelberg, Victoria 3084, Australia
[b] The Mental Health Research Institute of Victoria, 135 Oak Street, Parkville, Victoria 3052, Australia
[c] Department of Medicine, Austin Health, Victoria 3084, Australia
* Corresponding author. Department of Nuclear Medicine and Centre for PET, Austin Health, 145 Studley Road, Heidelberg, Victoria 3084, Australia.
E-mail address: villemagne@petnm.unimelb.edu.au

PET Clin 5 (2010) 33–53
doi:10.1016/j.cpet.2009.12.008
1556-8598/10/$ – see front matter

activities of daily living, and the exclusion of other diseases.[24] A period of up to 5 years of prodromal decline in cognition, known as mild cognitive impairment (MCI), usually precedes the formal diagnosis of AD.[25–27] About 40% to 60% of carefully characterized subjects with MCI will subsequently progress to meet criteria for AD over a 3- to 4-year period.[28,29]

At this point there is no cure for AD, but a growing understanding of the molecular mechanisms of Aβ formation, degradation, and neurotoxicity is being translated into new therapeutic approaches.[1,23,30] Palliative treatment regimens involve the use of acetylcholinesterase inhibitors and glutamatergic agents.[30] The most promising approaches focus on reducing Aβ formation through secretase inhibitors or on increasing the removal of Aβ by immunotherapy or metal-protein attenuating compounds (MPAC) aimed at removing or blocking the formation of Aβ oligomers, inhibiting neurotoxicity.[30,31]

Although AD is the most common cause of dementia in the elderly, postmortem studies have found dementia with Lewy Bodies (DLB) to account for 20% of cases.[32] Although the pathologic hallmark of DLB is the finding of cortical Lewy bodies, the majority of cases also show extensive cortical Aβ deposition.[32] The contribution of Aβ to the development of DLB is unclear. Postmortem histopathological studies of DLB have identified that the majority of patients have cortical Aβ deposits with characteristics in a distribution similar to AD patients. This condition may be described as "mixed" DLB/AD. So-called pure DLB is much less common, and it is not clear if the clinical characteristics and prognosis differ from the mixed pathology cases.[33] Cortical Aβ is not present in cognitively intact Parkinson disease (PD) patients; it may be present, however, when PD patients develop dementia along with Lewy bodies in the neocortex. The cortical Aβ deposits in PD with dementia are associated with extensive α-synuclein lesions and higher levels of insoluble α-synuclein, suggesting that Aβ enhances the development of cortical α-synuclein lesions.[34] These data suggest a central role for Aβ in several types of dementia.

Frontotemporal lobe degeneration (FTLD) accounts for about 20% of cases of dementia in postmortem studies.[35] Neuropathologically there is atrophy of frontal and temporal lobes, severe neuronal loss, gray and white matter gliosis, and superficial laminar spongiosis, with absence of amyloid aggregates. In many cases there is accumulation of insoluble tau within neurons and glia,[36,37] whereas other cases are characterized by the presence of misfolded proteins that do not form amyloid deposits, such as TDP-43.[38,39]

Molecular neuroimaging techniques such as PET have been used for the in vivo assessment of molecular processes at their sites of action, permitting detection of subtle pathophysiological changes in the brain at asymptomatic stages, when there is no evidence of anatomic changes on computed tomography (CT) or magnetic resonance (MR) imaging.[40–43] The development of molecular imaging methods for noninvasively assessing disease-specific traits such as Aβ burden in AD is allowing early diagnosis at presymptomatic stages and more accurate differential diagnosis as well as, when available, the evaluation and monitoring of disease-modifying therapy (**Box 1**).[1,44,45]

AMYLOID LIGANDS

Aβ plaques and NFT are the hallmark brain lesions of AD. These microscopic aggregates are still well beyond the resolution of conventional neuroimaging techniques used for the clinical evaluation of patients with AD. Selective tau imaging, for in vivo NFT quantification, is still in the early stages of development.[46–48] Because Aβ is at the center of AD pathogenesis, and given that several pharmacologic agents aimed at reducing Aβ levels in the brain are being developed and tested, many efforts are focused on generating radiotracers or agents that allow Aβ imaging in vivo.[49–51]

For a radiotracer to be useful as a neuroimaging Aβ probe, several key general properties are desirable: they should be lipophilic molecules that cross the blood-brain barrier (BBB) and preferably not be metabolized, while reversibly binding to Aβ in a specific and selective fashion.[45] Furthermore, low nonspecific binding to white matter is desirable (**Box 2**). Therapies, especially those targeting irreversible neurodegenerative processes, have a better chance to succeed if applied early, which is why early detection of the underlying pathologic process is so important. Aβ deposition usually

---

Box 1
Potential roles for Aβ imaging

- Accurate diagnosis of AD
- Prognosis of conversion to AD
- Early diagnosis of AD, allowing intervention when minimally impaired
- Investigate the spatial and temporal pattern of Aβ deposition and its relation to disease progression, cognitive decline, and other disease biomarkers
- Subject selection for anti-Aβ trials
- Monitor the effectiveness of anti-Aβ therapy
- Predict response to anti-Aβ therapy

Box 2
Ideal Aβ radiotracer

- Easily labeled with ^{18}F, ^{99m}Tc, [123]I
- Lipid soluble (crosses BBB)
- High affinity and selectivity for Aβ plaques
- Slow dissociation from binding site
- Rapidly cleared from blood
- Not metabolized
- Low nonspecific binding
- Provide quantitative and reproducible information about Aβ burden in the brain

starts at layers III and IV of the cortex,[52] and spill-over from high nonspecific binding in white matter might mask or reduce the ability to detect this early deposition.

Several compounds have been evaluated as potential Aβ probes. It has been known since the 1930s that Aβ plaques present in postmortem AD brain tissue can be stained for histologic examination with Congo red or Chrysamine-G. Klunk and colleagues[53–55] at the University of Pittsburgh developed numerous Congo red derivatives for potential use as in vivo Aβ probes, but these relatively large and acidic compounds' ability to cross the BBB was found to be marginal at best. A ^{11}C-labeled methoxy derivative of Congo red, methoxy-X04, was shown to have more favorable BBB penetration and fluorescent properties that allowed visualization of individual 1-μm Aβ plaques with multiphoton microscopy in PS1/APP transgenic mice.[56] Thioflavin T derivatives have shown even more favorable Aβ binding characteristics.[57–65] Synthesis and initial characterization of ^{125}I-bromostyrylbenzene (BSB) probes were described by Kung and colleagues[66–68] from the University of Pennsylvania, Philadelphia. Other BSB isomers were radiolabeled by the same group and their in vitro binding properties to postmortem AD tissues assessed.[69–71] All these compounds were found to strongly bind to Aβ amyloid plaques as assessed by fluorescent microscopy, but displayed low in vivo brain uptake. Furthermore, BSB was shown to not only bind to Aβ deposits but also to hyperphosphorylated tau in neurofibrillary tangles, neuropil threads, and a-synuclein, both in Lewy Bodies and related cytoplasmic inclusions found in multiple system atrophy.[72] New PET and single-photon emission CT (SPECT) compounds were further developed and characterized by the same group.[73–79]

Anti-Aβ monoclonal antibodies that bind to specific epitopes within Aβ fibrils have been developed and used in vitro in human brain tissue.[80,81]

Because antibodies are poorly delivered into the central nervous system when administered peripherally, they have usually failed as tracers for in vivo brain imaging studies. Other groups have proposed using self-associating Aβ fragments,[82–84] anti-Aβ antibodies fragments,[85] and serum amyloid P and basic fibroblast growth factor and Aβ tracers.[86]

Almost a decade after unsuccessful trials with anti-Aβ antibodies,[80] amyloid imaging came to fruition with the first report of successful imaging in an AD patient with ^{18}F-FDDNP, a tracer characterized for binding both plaques and NFT.[87] Since then, human amyloid imaging studies have been conducted in AD patients, normal controls, and patients with other dementias using ^{11}C-PiB (Pittsburgh compound B),[88] ^{11}C-SB13,[89] ^{11}C-ST1859,[90] ^{11}C-BF227,[91] ^{11}C-AZD2138,[92] ^{18}F-BAY94-91772,[93] ^{18}F-GE067,[94] and ^{18}F-AV-45.[95] with PET and with ^{123}I-CQ[96] and ^{123}I-IMPY[97] (6-iodo-2-(4'-dimethylamino)-phenyl-imidazo[1,2-a]pyridine) using SPECT (**Fig. 1**).

Whereas all of the aforementioned tracers bind with varying degrees of success to Aβ fibrils and brain homogenates of AD patients, Congo Red and Thioflavin T—and some of their derivatives—have recently been shown to also bind to the soluble oligomeric forms of Aβ.[98] On the other hand, Aβ soluble species represent less than 1% of the total brain Aβ,[16] and the reported affinity of PiB for these soluble oligomers seems to be significantly lower than for Aβ fibrils.[98] Concurring with these findings, a recent report described a patient with a novel APP mutation where Aβ does not fibrilize remaining in an oligomeric state, in whom PiB PET scans showed some degree of cortical retention, though much lower than the one usually observed in sporadic AD.[99] Until highly selective radiotracers are developed to bind the Aβ soluble species, the contribution of these oligomers to the amyloid imaging PET signal in sporadic AD from tracers such as ^{11}C-PiB is considered to be negligible.[44]

To test compounds that could have more widespread application, preliminary studies with SPECT Aβ radiotracers ^{123}I-CQ[96] and ^{123}I-IMPY[97] (see **Fig. 1**) showed limited utility for the evaluation of Aβ burden in AD, although ^{123}I-IMPY might be useful in the evaluation of transmissible spongiform encephalopathies.[100] New SPECT radiotracers labeled with ^{123}I or those that could be potentially labeled with ^{99m}Tc are being evaluated.[101–104] Most PET amyloid imaging agents have been shown to display nanomolar affinity for Aβ, but only a few of these agents have found their way into human clinical trials (see **Fig. 1**).

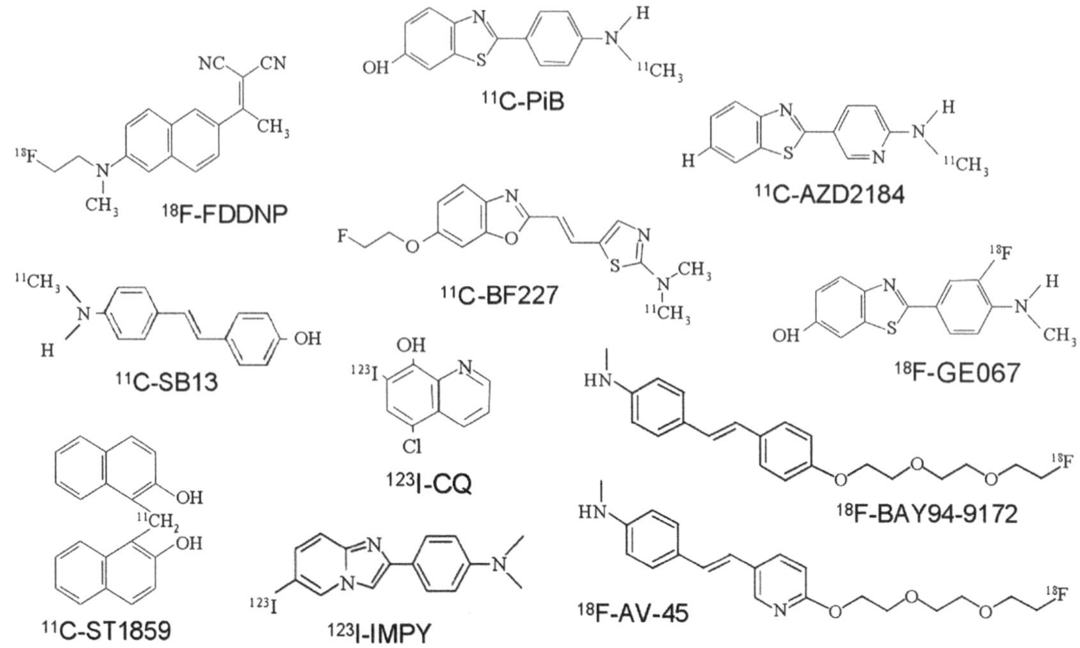

Fig. 1. Amyloid ligands. Chemical structure of amyloid ligands that have been used in clinical studies.

^{11}C Labeled Radiotracers

^{11}C-PiB

^{11}C-PiB (see Fig. 1), the most successful and widely used of the currently available amyloid tracers, has been shown to possess high affinity for fibrillar Aβ.[51,63,65,105–107] In vitro studies with ^{3}H-PiB of high specific activity demonstrated 2 binding sites for PiB in brain homogenates and Aβ$_{1-42}$ fibrils.[108] Recent studies have shown that PiB binds with high affinity to the N-terminally truncated and modified Aβ and AβN3-pyroglutamate species in senile plaques.[109] In vitro assessment of ^{3}H-PiB binding to white matter homogenates failed to show any specific binding.[110] PiB is a derivative of Thioflavin T, a fluorescent dye commonly used to assess fibrilization into β-sheet conformation,[111] and as such PiB has been shown to bind to a range of additional Aβ-containing lesions including diffuse plaques and cerebrovascular amyloid angiopathy (CAA),[112] as well as to Aβ oligomers—albeit with lower affinity[98]—or other misfolded proteins with a similar β-sheet secondary structure such as α-synuclein[113,114] and tau.[112,115] This finding is important, particularly because AD has been described as a "triple brain amyloidosis."[116] Furthermore, these studies have shown that, at the concentrations achieved during a PET examination, ^{11}C-PiB cortical retention in AD or DLB primarily reflects Aβ-related cerebral amyloidosis and not binding to Lewy bodies or NFT.[64,112,113,115]

^{11}C-SB13

The stilbene derivative, ^{11}C-SB13 (see Fig. 1) was evaluated in 5 AD patients and 6 age-matched healthy controls (HC) and compared with ^{11}C-PiB,[89] after in vitro binding studies with ^{3}H-SB-13 demonstrated a K_d of 2.4 nM.[117] The study showed that ^{11}C-SB13 could differentiate between AD and controls but showed lower effect size values when compared with ^{11}C-PiB.

^{11}C-ST1859

A preliminary study with the antiamyloid agent ^{11}C-ST1859 (see Fig. 1) revealed small differences in radiotracer retention between 9 AD patients and 3 HC, showing that the biodistribution and specificity of therapeutic agents can be assessed with PET.[90]

^{11}C-BF227

Benzoxazole derivatives are also promising tools as Aβ imaging tracers.[118] In vitro binding studies with BF-227 demonstrated a K_i value of 4.3 nM for the compound to Aβ$_{1-42}$ fibrils.[119] A PET study using ^{11}C-BF-227 (see Fig. 1) showed that AD patients were clearly distinguishable from age-matched controls, with AD patients displaying significantly higher tracer retention in the cerebral cortex than controls.[91] Regional parametric analysis of the images further demonstrated a higher retention of ^{11}C-BF-227 in the posterior association cortex in AD patients. In a similar fashion to most amyloid tracers, BF-227 also binds to other misfolded proteins with a secondary β-sheet structure such as α-synuclein.[120] A preliminary study in transmissible spongiform encephalopathies has shown that ^{11}C-BF-227 might be able to distinguish between Gerstmann-Straussler-Scheinker disease and sporadic Creutzfeldt-Jakob disease (CJD).[121]

[11]C-AZD2138

An appealing feature of this novel radiotracer (see **Fig. 1**) is that besides its reversible binding it displays very low nonspecific binding to white matter, showing a strong potential as an amyloid tracer.[92,122] Furthermore, an F-18 derivative has recently entered phase 2 studies (see later discussion).

[18]F-Labeled Radiotracers

Unfortunately, the 20-minute radioactive decay half-life of ^{11}C limits the use of ^{11}C radiotracers to centers with an on-site cyclotron and ^{11}C radiochemistry expertise. Access to ^{11}C-labeled radiotracers consequently is restricted and the high cost of studies is prohibitive for routine clinical use. To overcome these limitations, an Aβ imaging tracer labeled with ^{18}F was required. The 110-minute radioactive decay half-life of ^{18}F permits centralized production and regional distribution as currently practiced worldwide in the supply of ^{18}F-fluorodeoxyglucose (FDG) for clinical use. Several of the novel amyloid ligands are labeled with [18]F.

^{18}F-FDDNP

A marked progression in the development of amyloid-imaging tracers was the synthesis and characterization by Barrio and colleagues[123–125] of a very lipophilic radiofluorinated 6-dialkylamino-2-naphthyethylidene derivative that presents nanomolar affinity to Aβ fibrils. ^{18}F-FDDNP is reported to bind both the extracellular Aβ plaques and the intracellular NFT in AD[87] while also binding to prion plaques from CJD.[126] ^{18}F-FDDNP was used to obtain the first human PET images of Aβ in an 82-year-old woman with AD. In brief, ^{18}F-FDDNP showed a differential clearance, being slower from areas of plaque deposition such as the hippocampus, as pathologically confirmed later at postmortem examination.[123] In a follow-up study, AD patients again demonstrated higher accumulation and slower clearance of ^{18}F-FDDNP than controls in brain areas such as the hippocampus.[87] Retention time of ^{18}F-FDDNP in these brain regions was correlated with lower memory performance scores in patients with AD.[127] These findings were further confirmed in a larger series where AD and MCI participants were successfully

differentiated from those with no cognitive impairment.[128] However, the analysis required a 2-hour continuous scan and only demonstrated 9% higher cortical uptake in AD. Direct comparison of ^{18}F-FDDNP with ^{11}C-PiB in monkeys[129] and in human subjects showed a very limited dynamic range of ^{18}F-FDDNP.[130,131] Of note, ^{18}F-FDDNP still remains the only tracer showing retention in the medial temporal cortex of AD patients, suggesting higher binding affinity of FDDNP to NFT than to Aβ.[131] However, in vitro evaluation of FDDNP in concentrations similar to those achieved during a PET scan showed limited binding to both NFT and Aβ plaques.[132]

^{18}F-BAY94-9172

^{18}F-BAY94-9172 (also known as Florbetaben) (see **Fig. 1**) has been shown to bind avidly to neuritic and diffuse amyloid plaques and to CAA. BAY94-9172 was found to bind with high affinity to Aβ in brain homogenates and selectively labeled Aβ plaques in AD tissue sections.[133] At tracer concentrations achieved during human PET studies, BAY94-9172 did not show binding to postmortem cortex from subjects with FTLD. After injection into Tg2576 transgenic mice, ex vivo brain sections showed localization of ^{18}F-BAY94-9172 in regions with Aβ plaques, as confirmed by thioflavin binding.[134] In human studies, ^{18}F-BAY94-9172 neocortical retention was higher at 90 minutes post injection in all AD subjects compared with age-matched controls and FTLD patients, with binding matching the reported postmortem distribution of Aβ plaques.[93] Recently completed phase 2 clinical studies further confirmed these results.

^{18}F-AV45

As was ^{18}F-BAY94-9172, this stilbene derivative was developed by Kung's group[134] at the University of Pennsylvania (see **Fig. 1**). The most salient feature of this tracer is its rapid reversible binding characteristics, allowing scanning subjects only at 45 to 50 minutes after injection.[95] Several studies have used ^{18}F-AV-45 (Florpiramine) and a multicenter phase 2 study in AD, MCI, and HC subjects have just been completed, showing the ability of ^{18}F-AV-45 to discriminate between AD and age-matched controls.[135,136] ^{18}F-AV-45 is widely available in more than 40 centers in the United States and is being used in a large number of therapeutic clinical trials around the world.

^{18}F-GE067

Another fluorinated tracer that has just completed phase II studies is ^{18}F-GE067.[94,137] The new studies with ^{18}F-GE067 (Flutemetamol) (see **Fig. 1**) have shown that it can differentiate between AD and controls and that it displays equivalent regional distribution than ^{11}C-PiB.[138,139]

^{18}F-AZD4694

Also developed at Astra-Zeneca as ^{11}C-AZD2138, the most salient feature of ^{18}F-AZD4694 is the low nonspecific binding to white matter, suggesting it might be helpful for the detection of small Aβ cortical deposits at very early stages of the disease process.[140]

AMYLOID IMAGING IN DEMENTIA

Clinical imaging studies with amyloid radiotracers are providing quantitative information on Aβ burden in vivo, leading to new insights into Aβ deposition in the brain and facilitating research of neurodegenerative diseases in which Aβ may play a role.[1,31,44,88,141] Most of the amyloid imaging studies worldwide had been conducted using ^{11}C-PiB, the most successful and widespread amyloid imaging agent to date.

On visual inspection, cortical retention of ^{11}C-PiB, regardless of disease severity, is markedly elevated in AD,[88,141–143] while being generally lower and more variable in DLB, probably reflecting a larger spectrum of Aβ deposition.[141,144,145] In AD, ^{11}C-PiB retention is highest in frontal, cingulate, precuneus, striatum, parietal, and lateral temporal cortex (**Fig. 2**). Occipital cortex, sensorimotor cortex, and mesial temporal cortex are usually less affected (see **Fig. 2**). With the exception of ^{18}F-FDDNP, which shows high retention in the mesial temporal cortex, a similar pattern of retention in AD is observed with most ^{11}C and ^{18}F amyloid ligands. ^{11}C-PiB binds reversibly, with fastest clearance from the cerebellar cortex and slowest from white matter,[88,105,141,146] whereas absence of neuritic Aβ plaques in the cerebellar cortex of AD patients[115,147] is reflected in a similar clearance from this region in all groups,[105,141,146] with the exception of familial AD cases[148,149] or prion diseases like CJD (**Fig. 3**).[150,151] No significant ^{11}C-PiB cortical retention was observed in a preliminary report on PD patients,[152] nor when it was used to discriminate between AD, PD, DLB, and PD with dementia (see **Fig. 3**)[144,145,153,154] ^{11}C-PiB-PET has also facilitated differential diagnosis of dementia in patients with atypical onset of dementia who

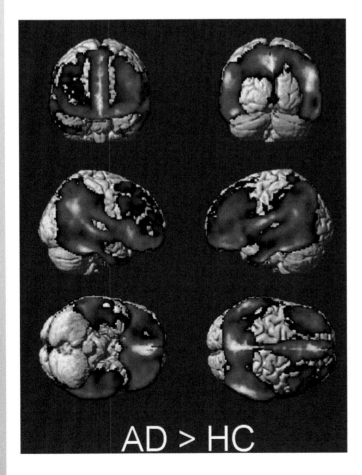

Fig. 2. Typical pattern of ^{11}C-PiB retention in AD. SPM projection of regions with significant higher (uncorrected $P<.0001$) ^{11}C-PiB retention in AD patients compared with control subjects (yellow = most significant difference). ^{11}C-PiB retention is observed in frontal, temporal, and parietal cortices as well as in the posterior cingulate/precuneus areas, with relative sparing of occipital and sensorimotor cortex.

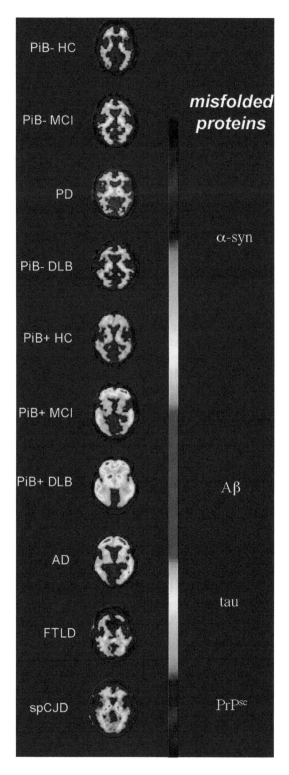

Fig. 3. Amyloid imaging in aging and dementia. Representative transaxial ^{11}C-PiB images 40 to 70 minutes post injection along the spectrum of some of the misfolded proteins associated with neurodegenerative diseases, encompassing the different patterns of ^{11}C-PiB retention in the brain, with (from top to bottom) a 73-year-old healthy PiB-negative control (PiB– HC) subject (MMSE 30), an 83-year-old PiB-negative subject with mild cognitive impairment (PiB– MCI) (MMSE 28), a 61-year-old PiB-negative Parkinson disease (PD) patient (MMSE 27), a 69-year-old PiB-negative patient with dementia with Lewy Bodies (DLB; MMSE 24), a 77-year-old PiB-positive healthy control (PiB+ HC) subject (MMSE 28), an 82-year-old PiB-positive subject with mild cognitive impairment (PiB+ MCI) (MMSE 28), a 78-year-old PiB-positive DLB patient (PiB+ DLB) (MMSE 19), a 76-year-old Alzheimer's disease (AD) patient (MMSE 21), a 59-year-old patient with frontotemporal lobe degeneration (FTLD; MMSE 20), and a 59-year-old PiB-negative patient with confirmed sporadic Creutzfeldt-Jakob disease (spCJD). PET images show clear differences when comparing cortical PiB retention in PiB-negative HC, MCI, PD, spCJD, and FTLD with PiB-positive HC, MCI, DLB, or AD patients. Only nonspecific PiB binding in white matter is observed in PiB-negative HC, MCI, PD, spCJD, and FTLD compared with PiB binding in cortical areas of AD and DLB patients. All images are scaled to the same standardized maximum uptake value ratio.

presented with provisional diagnosis of either progressive nonfluent aphasia—considered by many as a variant of FTLD—or posterior cortical atrophy, respectively.[155]

In a similar way to most of the available amyloid imaging tracers, quantitative and visual assessment of PET images present a pattern of ^{11}C-PiB retention that seems to replicate the sequence of Aβ deposition found at autopsy,[156,157] with initial deposition in orbitofrontal cortex and gyrus rectus, followed by the cingulate gyrus and precuneus, the remaining prefrontal cortex and lateral temporal cortex, and finally to the parietal cortex. The regional retention of ^{11}C-PiB reflects the regional density of Aβ plaques, as reported at autopsy,[115,158] with a higher plaque density in the frontal cortex than in hippocampus, consistent with previous neuropathological[159] and PiB PET reports.[141,160]

[11]C-PiB retention is also elevated in subjects diagnosed with CAA,[161] showing a similar distribution to AD and DLB cases.[141,144,145] There is usually no cortical ^{11}C-PiB retention in patients with clinical diagnosis of FTLD,[141,162–165] whereas analysis of ^{11}C-PiB binding in subjects diagnosed with MCI, a condition that progresses to AD at a rate of approximately 15% per year,[29,166] has revealed 2 distinct ^{11}C-PiB retention patterns (see **Fig. 3**). About 60% of MCI cases show cortical ^{11}C-PiB binding similar in distribution and sometimes in degree to AD, while the rest exhibit little or no cortical ^{11}C-PiB retention, similar to HC (see **Fig. 3**).[105,142,167,168]

Of note, about 25% to 35% of asymptomatic age-matched HC present with cortical ^{11}C-PiB retention, predominantly in the prefrontal and posterior cingulate/precuneus regions (see **Fig. 3**).[141,143,169,170] These findings are in agreement with postmortem reports that at least 30% of nondemented older individuals older than 75 years have amyloid plaques, with deposits occurring well before the onset of dementia.[171–174] The retention of ^{11}C-PiB in HC correlates with subtle memory impairment and a greater risk of cognitive decline,[143,168,169] likely to represent what has been termed preclinical AD,[175–178] and this group might comprise those who will benefit the most from therapies aimed at reducing or eliminating Aβ from the brain before irreversible neuronal or synaptic loss occurs.

AMYLOID IMAGING AND OTHER MARKERS OF DISEASE

In vivo amyloid imaging is not only helping elucidate the relation between Aβ deposition and cognition but is also allowing researchers to define

and refine its relationship with cerebrospinal fluid (CSF) and genetic biomarkers, as well as to establish the relation between Aβ deposition, neuropathology, brain atrophy, and glucose metabolism.

[11]C-PiB PET studies have shown not only a robust difference in ^{11}C-PiB retention between AD patients and age-matched controls,[88,141,179] but also inverse correlations with decreased CSF Aβ$_{42}$[180–182] and cerebral atrophy.[183–186] Amyloid imaging data concur both with postmortem reports on the regional density and sequence of Aβ deposition.[156,157,159] These data also agree with reports that these neuropathological changes precede the clinical expression of AD by many years,[178,187] reflected in the large percentage of cognitively unimpaired individuals with significant ^{11}C-PiB retention in the brain.[143,168–170] Despite a strong inverse correlation between PiB and FDG in temporal, parietal, and posterior cingulate cortex, the correlation is not present in the frontal lobe or hippocampus.[88,188,189] Visual assessment of PET images by clinicians blinded to the diagnoses demonstrated that ^{11}C-PiB was more accurate than FDG in distinguishing AD from HC.[190]

To date, the only consistent genetic marker for both the early-onset (familial) and late-onset (nonfamilial) forms of AD is the polymorphism of the ApoE allele on chromosome 19.[191] ApoE ε4 is the primary genetic risk factor associated with sporadic AD, and its presence is thought to result in an earlier age of onset.[192,193] Examination of ApoE ε4 allele status revealed that, independent of clinical classification, ε4 carriers present with significantly higher ^{11}C-PiB binding than non-ε4 carriers, further emphasizing the crucial role that ApoE plays in the metabolism of Aβ.[31,141,194] Both symptomatic and asymptomatic individuals with mutations within the APP or presenilin 1 (PS1) genes associated with familial AD present with very high PiB retention in the caudate nuclei and the posterior cingulate/precuneus and, to a lesser degree, in prefrontal and temporal cortices, retention that seems to be independent of mutation type or disease severity.[148,149,195]

To date, the relationship between Aβ deposition and the development of clinical symptoms is not fully understood. Although Aβ burden as assessed by PiB-PET does not correlate with measures of memory impairment in AD, it does correlate with memory impairment in MCI[142,168,186] and healthy older subjects.[168,169] It is interesting that 60% to 80% of the subjects classified as nonamnestic MCI do not show significant ^{11}C-PiB retention in the brain.[168,196] In contrast, 60% to 80% of amnestic MCI subjects were shown to have significant ^{11}C-PiB retention in the brain.[168,196,197] The observations that PiB retention in nondemented individuals relates to episodic memory impairment, one of the earliest clinical symptoms of AD, suggests that Aβ deposition is not part of normal ageing, and supports the hypothesis that Aβ deposition occurs well before the onset of symptoms and is likely to represent preclinical AD. The relation between the regional pattern of ^{11}C-PiB retention and its potential relation to cognition merits further comments. Multimodality studies in early AD have shown Aβ deposition in cortical regions that are associated with memory retrieval in young adults.[198] This Aβ deposition pattern has been associated with the anatomy of the "default network," a specific, anatomically defined brain system responsible for internal modes of cognition, such as self-reflection processes, conscious resting state, or episodic memory retrieval.[199,200] It has been proposed that deficits or disruption of the default activity in these cortical regions might predispose certain people to AD-related changes.[198]

Whereas one report of a 2-year follow-up study in AD patients showed that despite some participants presenting cognitive decline and increased FDG hypometabolism there was stable or even decreased ^{11}C-PiB binding,[201] another 1-year follow-up study on larger series including HC, MCI and AD subjects showed small increases in Aβ burden, with cognitive decline being associated with measures of brain atrophy and not with Aβ deposition.[202] These findings, in addition to the evidence of Aβ deposition in a high percentage of MCI and asymptomatic HC, suggest that Aβ is an early and necessary, though not sufficient, cause for cognitive decline in AD.[169] Perhaps specific in vivo tau imaging will help elucidate or bridge the gap between Aβ deposition and the persistent decline in cognitive function observed in AD. Ongoing large longitudinal studies including both structural and amyloid neuroimaging studies as well as genetic and biochemical biomarkers will permit a better understanding of the role and relevance of Aβ deposition in elderly controls and MCI subjects.[203,204]

The observed dissociation between Aβ deposition and measures of cognition, synaptic activity, and neurodegeneration in AD points toward other mechanisms likely triggered by β deposition such as NFT formation, synaptic failure, and eventually neuronal loss. Therefore, as stated earlier, β deposition is an early and necessary, although not sufficient cause for cognitive impairment in AD.[169] The evidence points to the fact that Aβ toxicity in the form of oligomers and Aβ deposition in the form of aggregates precede by many years the appearance of clinical symptoms.[174,178] These neurotoxic processes eventually lead to synaptic and neuronal loss, manifested as brain atrophy, glucose hypometabolism, and cognitive impairment.[186,202,205–207] Therefore, it is highly likely that PiB retention in nondemented individuals reflects preclinical AD.[141,143,169] As previously suggested,[169] this may be associated or attributed to a different susceptibility/vulnerability to Aβ, at both a cellular/regional level—frontal neurons seems to be more resistant to Aβ toxicity than hippocampal neurons[208–210]—as well as at an individual or personal level, due either to a particular cognitive reserve,[211–214] differences in Aβ conformation affecting toxicity or PiB binding,[106,215–218] or because an idiosyncratic threshold must be exceeded for synaptic failure and neuronal death to ensue.[207] These factors would help explain why some older individuals with a significant Aβ burden are cognitively unimpaired, whereas others with lower Aβ burden and no genetic predisposing factors have already developed the full clinical AD phenotype.

SPECIFIC BIOMARKERS OF DISEASE

The clinical diagnosis of AD is typically based on progressive cognitive impairments while excluding other diseases. Clinical diagnosis of sporadic disease is challenging, however, often presenting mild and nonspecific symptoms attributable to diverse and overlapping pathology presenting similar phenotypes. Confirmation of diagnosis of AD still relies on autopsy. Although clinical criteria, together with current structural neuroimaging techniques (CT or MR imaging), are sufficiently sensitive and specific for the diagnosis of AD at the mid to late stages of the disease, they are focused on nonspecific features derived mainly from neuronal loss and atrophy, which are late features in the progression of the disease and may be secondary to the basic functional alteration. The neurodegenerative process usually begins decades before symptoms are evident, making early identification based on structural neuroimaging difficult. This situation in turn precludes early intervention with disease-modifying medications during the presymptomatic period, which by arresting neuronal loss would presumably achieve the maximum benefits of such therapies.

Therefore, a change in the diagnostic paradigm is needed, whereby diagnosis moves away from identification of signs and symptoms of neuronal failure—indicating that central compensatory mechanisms have been exhausted and extensive synaptic and neuronal damage is present—to the noninvasive detection of specific biomarkers for particular traits underlying the pathologic process.[219] Given the complexity and sometimes overlapping characteristics of these disorders, and despite recent advances in molecular neurosciences, it is unlikely that a single biomarker will be able to provide the diagnostic certainty required for the early detection of neurodegenerative diseases like AD, especially for the identification of at-risk individuals before the development of the typical phenotype. Therefore, a multimodality approach combining biochemical and neuroimaging methods is warranted.[220]

Valid biomarkers are important as they can be used to identify the risk of developing a disease (antecedent biomarkers), aid in identifying disease (diagnostic biomarkers), assess disease evolution (progression biomarkers), or predict future disease course, including response to therapy (prognostic biomarkers). While neuropsychological evaluation, CSF assessment of Aβ and tau, and structural and molecular neuroimaging (both FDG and amyloid imaging) are all good diagnostic biomarkers for AD, evaluation of the data available to date suggests that amyloid imaging and CSF assessments are good antecedent biomarkers at the prodromal stages of the disease.[142,197,221–223] On the other hand, given the small increases observed over time in Aβ burden and the dissociation between Aβ burden and measures of cognition, brain atrophy, or glucose metabolism observed in AD, it seems that amyloid imaging might not be the best approach to monitor disease evolution. In contrast, structural neuroimaging, FDG, and neuropsychological evaluation seem to be excellent biomarkers of disease progression.[184,224,225]

Regarding prognostic biomarkers, a review of the literature shows that quantification of $A\beta_{1-42}$, total tau and p-tau in CSF, FDG, and a long list of assessment of brain atrophy and white matter hyperintensities with MR imaging have all been proposed as predictors of conversion to AD.[226–231] Besides the inverse correlation between $A\beta_{1-42}$ in CSF and Aβ burden in the brain as measured by PiB PET,[181] CSF tau/$A\beta_{1-42}$ ratios,[180] CSF $A\beta_{1-42}$/$A\beta_{1-40}$ ratios,[222] or assessment of C-terminal truncated Aβ peptides in CSF[221] show promise as predictors of future cognitive decline in nondemented individuals. It has been reported that faster rates of hippocampal and global brain atrophy are associated with cognitive decline.[224,232] However, the requirement of serial MR imaging, plus the significant overlap between those who cognitively decline and those who do not, indicates that it is unlikely that it will be able to provide prognostic information.[227,232] In addition, atrophy is a relatively late feature of the disease reflecting neurodegeneration, strongly suggesting that this approach might not be the most sensitive to predict cognitive decline. Due to its high sensitivity for detecting temporoparietal hypometabolism, FDG-PET has been proposed to improve diagnostic and prognostic accuracy in patients with probable AD.[233–235] To date, FDG-PET is the neuroimaging technique that has been shown to yield the highest prognostic value for providing a diagnosis of presymptomatic AD 2 or more years before the full dementia phenotype is manifested.[235–238] Posterior cingulate and temporoparietal hypometabolism were observed in MCI subjects when compared with controls, with additional bilateral hypometabolism in prefrontal areas in those MCI participants who progressed to probable AD.[239] FDG predicted conversion from MCI to AD with approximately 90% sensitivity and specificity, with either of them being 100% if combined with ApoE status.[240] While longitudinal studies will further clarify the role of

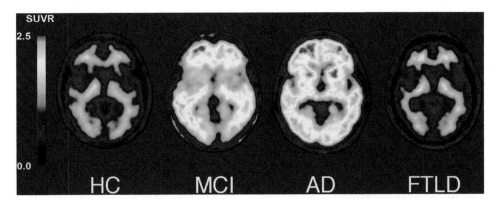

Fig. 4. Amyloid imaging with ^{18}F-BAY94-9172. Representative transaxial PET images obtained 90 to 120 minutes post injection of 300 MBq ^{18}F-BAY94-9172 in a healthy control (HC), a participant classified as mild cognitive impaired (MCI), one subject with Alzheimer's disease (AD), and one subject with frontotemporal lobar degeneration (FTLD). There is cortical binding in frontal, posterior cingulate/precuneus, and lateral temporal areas, with relative sparing of occipital and sensori-motor cortex in the MCI and AD subjects. In contrast, there is no cortical binding in the HC or FTLD subjects.

amyloid imaging in predicting conversion from MCI to AD,[142,197] one of the most important conclusions to be drawn from all these studies evaluating Aβ deposition in the brain is that the likelihood of developing AD in a cognitively unimpaired subject with a negative amyloid imaging scan is extremely low.

When antiamyloid therapies become available, amyloid imaging should allow not only assessment of eligibility of adequate candidates but also monitoring of such therapies, while also permitting its evaluation as a potential predictor of treatment response. In the meantime, amyloid imaging is well suited for subject selection and monitoring efficacy in antiamyloid therapy trials, aiding in reducing sample size and minimizing cost while maximizing outcomes.

SUMMARY

The introduction of radiotracers for the noninvasive in vivo quantification of Aβ in the brain has revolutionized the approach to the evaluation of AD. Frank and colleagues[241] proposed that an ideal biomarker for AD should be disease-specific and noninvasive, with sensitivity and specificity of more than 80%. Amyloid imaging fulfills these criteria. Aβ burden as measured by PET matches histopathological reports of Aβ distribution in aging and dementia, seems to be more accurate than FDG for the diagnosis of AD, and is an excellent aid in the differential diagnosis of AD from FTLD. ApoE ε4 status is associated with higher Aβ burden. As new treatments in clinical trials are

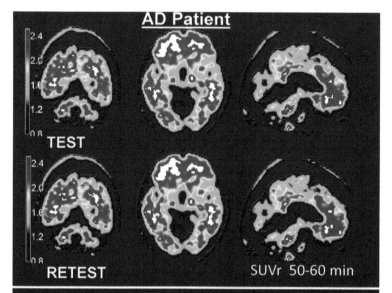

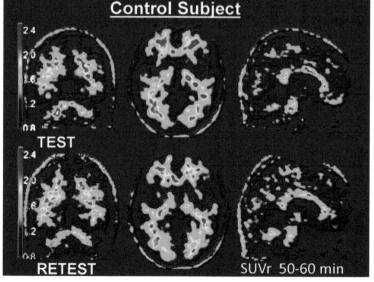

Fig. 5. Amyloid imaging with ^{18}F-AV-45. Representative coronal (*left column*), transaxial (*middle column*), and sagittal (*right column*) 10-minute PET images, acquired 50 minutes following iv injection of ^{18}F-AV-45 in an Alzheimer's disease (AD) patient (*top*) and a healthy control subject (*bottom*). The images show not only the ability of ^{18}F-AV-45 to differentiate AD patients from controls but also the high degree of reproducibility of the approach, with test-retest variance of 5%. (*Courtesy of* Dr Daniel Skovronsky, Avid Radiopharmaceuticals Inc, USA.)

aimed at preventing or slowing AD progression, either by preventing Aβ generation or deposition or increasing the clearance of Aβ, the role of imaging and quantifying Aβ burden in vivo is becoming increasingly crucial. Although these treatments are aimed at AD, the available data suggest that they may have value in other dementias such as DLB, where Aβ deposition is present.

Despite the development of promising new and reliable Aβ imaging ligands labeled with isotopes with longer radioactive half-lives **(Figs. 4–6)**,[93,95,137,140] population screening is unlikely to involve neuroimaging approaches and, despite the unreliability of plasma assays to date,[242] a simple blood test assessing central features of the disease, such as Aβ, as well as the use of near-infrared amyloid dyes[243,244] should soon be available to permit widespread screening of the at-risk population. On the other hand, molecular neuroimaging can provide highly accurate, reliable, and reproducible quantitative statements of Aβ burden, essential for therapeutic trial recruitment and for the evaluation of disease-specific treatments directed at removing Aβ.

Although Aβ burden as assessed by amyloid agents does not correlate with cognitive impairment in AD, it does correlate with memory impairment and the rate of memory decline in the aging population and MCI subjects. This correlation with memory impairment, one of the earliest symptoms of AD, suggests that Aβ deposition is not part of normal aging, supporting the hypothesis that Aβ deposition occurs well before the onset of symptoms and is likely to represent preclinical AD. Further longitudinal observations, coupled with different tracers to assess potential downstream effects of Aβ (eg, selective tau ligands) and biomarkers (eg, assessment of tau and Aβ in CSF and blood) are required not only to confirm this hypothesis but also to better elucidate the role of Aβ deposition in the course of AD.

REFERENCES

1. Masters CL, Cappai R, Barnham KJ, et al. Molecular mechanisms for Alzheimer's disease: implications for neuroimaging and therapeutics. J Neurochem 2006;97(6):1700–25.
2. Schneider J, Murray J, Banerjee S, et al. EUROCARE: a cross-national study of co-resident spouse carers for people with Alzheimer's disease: I—factors associated with carer burden. Int J Geriatr Psychiatry 1999;14(8):651–61.
3. Bennett DA. Part I. Epidemiology and public health impact of Alzheimer's disease. Dis Mon 2000; 46(10):657–65.
4. Johnson N, Davis T, Bosanquet N. The epidemic of Alzheimer's disease. How can we manage the costs? Pharmacoeconomics 2000;18(3):215–23.
5. Selkoe DJ. Alzheimer's disease is a synaptic failure. Science 2002;298(5594):789–91.
6. Masters CL. Neuropathology of Alzheimer's disease. In: Burns A, O'Brien J, Ames D, editors. Dementia. 3rd edition. London: Hodder Arnold; 2005. p. 393–407.
7. Masters CL, Beyreuther K. The neuropathology of Alzheimer's disease in the year 2005. In: Beal MF, Lang AE, Ludolph AC, editors. Neurodegenerative diseases: neurobiology, pathogenesis and therapeutics. Cambridge: Cambridge University Press; 2005. p. 433–40.
8. Jellinger K. Morphology of Alzheimer disease and related disorders. In: Maurer K, Riederer P, Beckmann H, editors. Alzheimer disease: epidemiology, neuropathology, neurochemistry, and clinics. Berlin: Springer-Verlag; 1990. p. 61–77.
9. Jellinger KA, Bancher C. Neuropathology of Alzheimer's disease: a critical update. J Neural Transm suppl 1998;54:77–95.

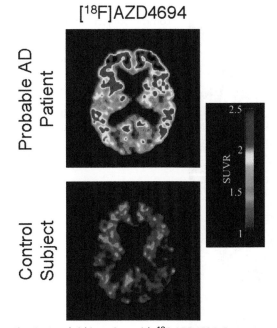

[18F]AZD4694

Probable AD Patient

Control Subject

SUVR
2.5
2
1.5
1

Fig. 6. Amyloid imaging with ^18F-AZD4694. Representative transaxial PET images obtained 20 to 40 minutes following intraventricular injection of ^18F-AZD4694 in an Alzheimer's disease (AD) patient (*top*) and a healthy control subject (*bottom*). The images show high cortical ^18F-AZD4694 retention in the AD patient. In comparison with other available radiotracers, ^18F-AZD4694 displays very low nonspecific binding to white matter. (*Courtesy of* Drs S. Svensson and Z. Cselényi, AstraZeneca R&D, Södertälje, Sweden.)

10. Michaelis ML, Dobrowsky RT, Li G. Tau neurofibrillary pathology and microtubule stability. J Mol Neurosci 2002;19(3):289–93.
11. Masters CL, Simms G, Weinman NA, et al. Amyloid plaque core protein in Alzheimer disease and down syndrome. Proc Natl Acad Sci U S A 1985; 82(12):4245–9.
12. Cappai R, White AR. Amyloid beta. Int J Biochem Cell Biol 1999;31(9):885–9.
13. Villemagne VL, Cappai R, Barnham KJ, et al. The Abeta centric pathway of Alzheimer's disease. In: Barrow CJ, Small BJ, editors. Abeta peptide and Alzheimer's disease. London: Springer-Verlag; 2006. p. 5–32.
14. Greenberg SM, Rebeck GW, Vonsattel JP, et al. Apolipoprotein E epsilon 4 and cerebral hemorrhage associated with amyloid angiopathy. Ann Neurol 1995;38(2):254–9.
15. Mega MS, Dinov ID, Porter V, et al. Metabolic patterns associated with the clinical response to galantamine therapy: a fludeoxyglucose F 18 positron emission tomographic study. Arch Neurol 2005;62(5):721–8.
16. McLean CA, Cherny RA, Fraser FW, et al. Soluble pool of Aβ amyloid as a determinant of severity of neurodegeneration in Alzheimer's disease. Ann Neurol 1999;46(6):860–6.
17. Arriagada PV, Growdon JH, Hedley-Whyte ET, et al. Neurofibrillary tangles but not senile plaques parallel duration and severity of Alzheimer's disease. Neurology 1992;42(3 Pt 1):631–9.
18. Lue LF, Kuo YM, Roher AE, et al. Soluble amyloid beta peptide concentration as a predictor of synaptic change in Alzheimer's disease. Am J Pathol 1999;155(3):853–62.
19. Wang J, Dickson DW, Trojanowski JQ, et al. The levels of soluble versus insoluble brain Aβ distinguish Alzheimer's disease from normal and pathologic aging. Exp Neurol 1999;158(2): 328–37.
20. Naslund J, Haroutunian V, Mohs R, et al. Correlation between elevated levels of amyloid beta-peptide in the brain and cognitive decline. JAMA 2000;283(12):1571–7.
21. McLean CA, Beyreuther K, Masters CL. Amyloid Abeta levels in Alzheimer's disease—a diagnostic tool and the key to understanding the natural history of Abeta? J Alzheimers Dis 2001;3(3): 305–12.
22. Walsh DM, Klyubin I, Fadeeva JV, et al. Naturally secreted oligomers of amyloid beta protein potently inhibit hippocampal long-term potentiation in vivo. Nature 2002;416(6880):535–9.
23. Walsh DM, Klyubin I, Shankar GM, et al. The role of cell-derived oligomers of Abeta in Alzheimer's disease and avenues for therapeutic intervention. Biochem Soc Trans 2005;33(Pt 5):1087–90.
24. McKhann G, Drachman D, Folstein M, et al. Clinical diagnosis of Alzheimer's disease: report of the NINCDS-ADRDA Work Group under the auspices of department of health and human services task force on Alzheimer's disease. Neurology 1984;34: 939–44.
25. Petersen RC. Mild cognitive impairment: current research and clinical implications. Semin Neurol 2007;27(1):22–31.
26. Petersen RC. Mild cognitive impairment: transition between aging and Alzheimer's disease. Neurologia 2000;15(3):93–101.
27. Petersen RC, Stevens JC, Ganguli M, et al. Practice parameter: early detection of dementia: mild cognitive impairment (an evidence-based review). Report of the quality standards subcommittee of the American academy of neurology. Neurology 2001;56(9):1133–42.
28. Petersen RC. Aging, mild cognitive impairment, and Alzheimer's disease. Neurol Clin 2000;18(4): 789–806.
29. Petersen RC, Smith GE, Waring SC, et al. Mild cognitive impairment: clinical characterization and outcome. Arch Neurol 1999;56(3):303–8.
30. Masters CL, Beyreuther K. Alzheimer's centennial legacy: prospects for rational therapeutic intervention targeting the Abeta amyloid pathway. Brain 2006;129(Pt 11):2823–39.
31. Villemagne VL, Ng S, Cappai R, et al. La Lunga Attesa: towards a molecular approach to neuroimaging and therapeutics in Alzheimer's disease. Neuroradiol J 2006;19:51–75.
32. McKeith IG, Dickson DW, Lowe J, et al. Diagnosis and management of dementia with Lewy bodies: third report of the DLB Consortium. Neurology 2005;65(12):1863–72.
33. Armstrong RA, Cairns NJ, Lantos PL. Beta-amyloid deposition in the temporal lobe of patients with dementia with Lewy bodies: comparison with non-demented cases and Alzheimer's disease. Dement Geriatr Cogn Disord 2000;11(4):187–92.
34. Pletnikova O, West N, Lee MK, et al. Abeta deposition is associated with enhanced cortical a-synuclein lesions in Lewy body diseases. Neurobiol Aging 2005;26:1183–92.
35. Mott RT, Dickson DW, Trojanowski JQ, et al. Neuropathologic, biochemical, and molecular characterization of the frontotemporal dementias. J Neuropathol Exp Neurol 2005;64(5):420–8.
36. Sergeant N, Delacourte A, Buee L. Tau protein as a differential biomarker of tauopathies. Biochim Biophys Acta 2005;1739(2–3):179–97.
37. Halliday G, Ng T, Rodriguez M, et al. Consensus neuropathological diagnosis of common dementia syndromes: testing and standardising the use of multiple diagnostic criteria. Acta Neuropathol (Berl) 2002;104(1):72–8.

38. Cairns NJ, Bigio EH, Mackenzie IR, et al. Neuro-pathologic diagnostic and nosologic criteria for frontotemporal lobar degeneration: consensus of the consortium for frontotemporal lobar degeneration. Acta Neuropathol 2007;114(1):5–22.

39. Neumann M, Kwong LK, Sampathu DM, et al. TDP-43 proteinopathy in frontotemporal lobar degeneration and amyotrophic lateral sclerosis: protein misfolding diseases without amyloidosis. Arch Neurol 2007;64(10):1388–94.

40. de Leon MJ, Convit A, DeSanti S, et al. Contribution of structural neuroimaging to the early diagnosis of Alzheimer's disease. Int Psychogeriatr 1997; 9(Suppl 1):183–90 [discussion: 247–52].

41. Dickerson BC, Goncharova I, Sullivan MP, et al. MRI-derived entorhinal and hippocampal atrophy in incipient and very mild Alzheimer's disease. Neurobiol Aging 2001;22(5):747–54.

42. Killiany RJ, Gomez-Isla T, Moss M, et al. Use of structural magnetic resonance imaging to predict who will get Alzheimer's disease. Ann Neurol 2000;47(4):430–9.

43. Xu Y, Jack CR Jr, O'Brien PC, et al. Usefulness of MRI measures of entorhinal cortex versus hippocampus in AD. Neurology 2000;54(9): 1760–7.

44. Mathis CA, Lopresti BJ, Klunk WE. Impact of amyloid imaging on drug development in Alzheimer's disease. Nucl Med Biol 2007;34(7):809–22.

45. Villemagne VL, Fodero-Tavoletti MT, Pike KE, et al. The ART of loss: Abeta imaging in the evaluation of Alzheimer's disease and other dementias. Mol Neurobiol 2008;38(1):1–15.

46. Okamura N, Suemoto T, Furumoto S, et al. Quinoline and benzimidazole derivatives: candidate probes for in vivo imaging of tau pathology in Alzheimer's disease. J Neurosci 2005;25(47):10857–62.

47. Ojida A, Sakamoto T, Inoue MA, et al. Fluorescent BODIPY-based Zn(II) complex as a molecular probe for selective detection of neurofibrillary tangles in the brains of Alzheimer's disease patients. J Am Chem Soc 2009;131(18):6543–8.

48. Maruyama M, Maeda J, Ji B, et al. In-vivo optical and PET detections of fibrillar tau lesions in a mouse model of tauopathies [abstract]. Alzheimers Dement 2009;55(4 Suppl 1):P209–10.

49. Sair HI, Doraiswamy PM, Petrella JR. In vivo amyloid imaging in Alzheimer's disease. Neuroradiology 2004;46(2):93–104.

50. Villemagne VL, Rowe CC, Macfarlane S, et al. Imaginem oblivionis: the prospects of neuroimaging for early detection of Alzheimer's disease. J Clin Neurosci 2005;12(3):221–30.

51. Mathis CA, Klunk WE, Price JC, et al. Imaging technology for neurodegenerative diseases: progress toward detection of specific pathologies. Arch Neurol 2005;62(2):196–200.

52. Thal DR, Rub U, Schultz C, et al. Sequence of Abeta-protein deposition in the human medial temporal lobe. J Neuropathol Exp Neurol 2000;59(8):733–48.

53. Link CD, Johnson CJ, Fonte V, et al. Visualization of fibrillar amyloid deposits in living, transgenic Caenorhabditis elegans animals using the sensitive amyloid dye, X-34. Neurobiol Aging 2001;22(2): 217–26.

54. Klunk WE, Debnath ML, Pettegrew JW. Development of small molecule probes for the beta-amyloid protein of Alzheimer's disease. Neurobiol Aging 1994;15(6):691–8.

55. Bacskai BJ, Klunk WE, Mathis CA, et al. Imaging amyloid-beta deposits in vivo. J Cereb Blood Flow Metab 2002;22(9):1035–41.

56. Klunk WE, Bacskai BJ, Mathis CA, et al. Imaging Aβ plaques in living transgenic mice with multiphoton microscopy and methoxy-X04, a systemically administered Congo red derivative. J Neuropathol Exp Neurol 2002;61(9):797–805.

57. Bacskai BJ, Hickey GA, Skoch J, et al. Four-dimensional multiphoton imaging of brain entry, amyloid binding, and clearance of an amyloid-beta ligand in transgenic mice. Proc Natl Acad Sci U S A 2003;100(21):12462–7.

58. Mathis CA, Wang Y, Holt DP, et al. Synthesis and evaluation of ^{11}C-labeled 6-substituted 2-arylbenzothiazoles as amyloid imaging agents. J Med Chem 2003;46(13):2740–54.

59. Wang Y, Klunk WE, Huang GF, et al. Synthesis and evaluation of 2-(3′-iodo-4′-aminophenyl)-6-hydroxybenzothiazole for in vivo quantitation of amyloid deposits in Alzheimer's disease. J Mol Neurosci 2002;19(1–2):11–6.

60. Wang Y, Mathis CA, Huang GF, et al. Effects of lipophilicity on the affinity and nonspecific binding of iodinated benzothiazole derivatives. J Mol Neurosci 2003;20(3):255–60.

61. Helmuth L. Long-awaited technique spots Alzheimer's toxin. Science 2002;297:752–3.

62. Mathis CA, Holt DP, Wang Y, et al. Lipophilic ^{11}C-labelled thioflavin-T analogues for imaging amyloid plaques in Alzheimer's disease. J. Labelled Cpd Radiopharm 2001;44(Suppl 1):S26–8.

63. Klunk WE, Wang Y, Huang GF, et al. Uncharged thioflavin-T derivatives bind to amyloid-beta protein with high affinity and readily enter the brain. Life Sci 2001;69(13):1471–84.

64. Klunk WE, Wang Y, Huang GF, et al. The binding of 2-(4′-methylaminophenyl)benzothiazole to postmortem brain homogenates is dominated by the amyloid component. J Neurosci 2003;23(6): 2086–92.

65. Mathis CA, Bacskai BJ, Kajdasz ST, et al. A lipophilic thioflavin-T derivative for positron emission tomography (PET) imaging of amyloid in brain. Bioorg Med Chem Lett 2002;12(3):295–8.

66. Zhuang ZP, Kung MP, Hou C, et al. Radioiodinated styrylbenzenes and thioflavins as probes for amyloid aggregates. J Med Chem 2001;44(12):1905–14.

67. Kung HF, Lee CW, Zhuang ZP, et al. Novel stilbenes as probes for amyloid plaques. J Am Chem Soc 2001;123(50):12740–1.

68. Skovronsky DM, Zhang B, Kung MP, et al. In vivo detection of amyloid plaques in a mouse model of Alzheimer's disease. Proc Natl Acad Sci U S A 2000;97(13):7609–14.

69. Kung MP, Hou C, Zhuang ZP, et al. Radioiodinated styrylbenzene derivatives as potential SPECT imaging agents for amyloid plaque detection in Alzheimer's disease. J Mol Neurosci 2002;19(1–2):7–10.

70. Zhuang ZP, Kung MP, Hou C, et al. IBOX(2-(4'-di-methylaminophenyl)-6-iodobenzoxazole): a ligand for imaging amyloid plaques in the brain. Nucl Med Biol 2001;28(8):887–94.

71. Lee CW, Zhuang ZP, Kung MP, et al. Isomerization of (Z, Z) to (E, E)1-bromo-2,5-bis-(3-hydroxycar-bonyl-4-hydroxy)styrylbenzene in strong base: probes for amyloid plaques in the brain. J Med Chem 2001;44(14):2270–5.

72. Schmidt ML, Schuck T, Sheridan S, et al. The fluorescent Congo red derivative, (trans, trans)-1-bromo-2,5-bis-(3-hydroxycarbonyl-4-hydroxy)styrylbenzene (BSB), labels diverse β-pleated sheet structures in postmortem human neurodegenerative disease brains. Am J Pathol 2001;159(3):937–43.

73. Zhuang ZP, Kung MP, Wilson A, et al. Structure-activity relationship of imidazo[1,2-a]pyridines as ligands for detecting beta-amyloid plaques in the brain. J Med Chem 2003;46(2):237–43.

74. Kung MP, Hou C, Zhuang ZP, et al. IMPY: an improved thioflavin-T derivative for in vivo labeling of beta-amyloid plaques. Brain Res Bull 2002;956(2):202–10.

75. Ono M, Kung MP, Hou C, et al. Benzofuran derivatives as Abeta-aggregate-specific imaging agents for Alzheimer's disease. Nucl Med Biol 2002;29(6):633–42.

76. Ono M, Wilson A, Nobrega J, et al. ^{11}C-labeled stilbene derivatives as Abeta-aggregate-specific PET imaging agents for Alzheimer's disease. Nucl Med Biol 2003;30(6):565–71.

77. Kung MP, Skovronsky DM, Hou C, et al. Detection of amyloid plaques by radioligands for Abeta40 and Abeta42: potential imaging agents in Alzheimer's patients. J Mol Neurosci 2003;20(1):15–24.

78. Kung MP, Zhuang ZP, Hou C, et al. Characterization of radioiodinated ligand binding to amyloid beta plaques. J Mol Neurosci 2003;20(3):249–54.

79. Lee CW, Kung MP, Hou C, et al. Dimethylamino-fluorenes: ligands for detecting beta-amyloid plaques in the brain. Nucl Med Biol 2003;30(6):573–80.

80. Majocha RE, Reno JM, Friedland RP, et al. Development of a monoclonal antibody specific for b/A4 amyloid in Alzheimer's disease brain for application to in vivo imaging of amyloid angiopathy. J Nucl Med 1992;33(12):2184–9.

81. Walker LC, Price DL, Voytko ML, et al. Labelling of cerebral amyloid in vivo with a monoclonal antibody. J Neuropathol Exp Neurol 1994;53(4):377–83.

82. Lee VM. Related Amyloid binding ligands as Alzheimer's disease therapies. Neurobiol Aging 2002;23(6):1039–42.

83. Marshall JR, Stimson ER, Ghilardi JR, et al. Noninvasive imaging of peripherally injected Alzheimer's disease type synthetic A beta amyloid in vivo. Bioconjug Chem 2002;13(2):276–84.

84. Kurihara A, Pardridge WM. Abeta(1-40) peptide radiopharmaceuticals for brain amyloid imaging: (111)In chelation, conjugation to poly(ethylene glycol)-biotin linkers, and autoradiography with Alzheimer's disease brain sections. Bioconjug Chem 2000;11(3):380–6.

85. Poduslo JF, Ramakrishnan M, Holasek SS, et al. In vivo targeting of antibody fragments to the nervous system for Alzheimer's disease immunotherapy and molecular imaging of amyloid plaques. J Neurochem 2007;102(2):420–33.

86. Shi J, Perry G, Berridge MS, et al. Labeling of cerebral amyloid beta deposits in vivo using intranasal basic fibroblast growth factor and serum amyloid P component in mice. J Nucl Med 2002;43(8):1044–51.

87. Shoghi-Jadid K, Small GW, Agdeppa ED, et al. Localization of neurofibrillary tangles and beta-amyloid plaques in the brains of living patients with Alzheimer disease. Am J Geriatr Psychiatry 2002;10(1):24–35.

88. Klunk WE, Engler H, Nordberg A, et al. Imaging brain amyloid in Alzheimer's disease with Pittsburgh Compound-B. Ann Neurol 2004;55(3):306–19.

89. Verhoeff NP, Wilson AA, Takeshita S, et al. In-vivo imaging of Alzheimer disease beta-amyloid with [11C]SB-13 PET. Am J Geriatr Psychiatry 2004;12(6):584–95.

90. Bauer M, Langer O, Dal-Bianco P, et al. A positron emission tomography microdosing study with a potential antiamyloid drug in healthy volunteers and patients with Alzheimer's disease. Clin Pharmacol Ther 2006;80(3):216–27.

91. Kudo Y, Okamura N, Furumoto S, et al. 2-(2-[2-Dimethylaminothiazol-5-yl]ethenyl)-6-(2-[fluoro]ethoxy)benzoxazole: a novel PET agent for in vivo detection of dense amyloid plaques in Alzheimer's disease patients. J Nucl Med 2007;48(4):553–61.

92. Nyberg S, Jonhagen ME, Cselenyi Z, et al. Detection of amyloid in Alzheimer's disease with positron

emission tomography using [(11)C]AZD2184. Eur J Nucl Med Mol Imaging 2009;36:1859–63.

93. Rowe CC, Ackerman U, Browne W, et al. Imaging of amyloid beta in Alzheimer's disease with (18)F-BAY94-9172, a novel PET tracer: proof of mechanism. Lancet Neurol 2008;7(2):129–35.

94. Serdons K, Terwinghe C, Vermaelen P, et al. Synthesis and evaluation of (18)F-labeled 2-phenyl-benzothiazoles as positron emission tomography imaging agents for amyloid plaques in Alzheimer's disease. J Med Chem 2009;52:7090–102.

95. Wong DF, Rosenberg P, Zhou Y, et al. In vivo imaging of amyloid deposition in Alzheimer's disease using the novel radioligand [F-18]AV-45 [abstract]. J Nucl Med 2008;49:214P.

96. Opazo C, Luza S, Villemagne VL, et al. Radioiodi-nated clioquinol as a biomarker for beta-amyloid:Zn complexes in Alzheimer's disease. Aging Cell 2006;5(1):69–79.

97. Newberg AB, Wintering NA, Plossl K, et al. Safety, biodistribution, and dosimetry of ^{123}I-IMPY: a novel amyloid plaque-imaging agent for the diagnosis of Alzheimer's disease. J Nucl Med 2006;47(5):748–54.

98. Maezawa I, Hong HS, Liu R, et al. Congo red and thioflavin-T analogs detect Abeta oligomers. J Neurochem 2008;104(2):457–68.

99. Tomiyama T, Nagata T, Shimada H, et al. A new amyloid beta variant favoring oligomerization in Alzheimer's-type dementia. Ann Neurol 2008; 63(3):377–87.

100. Song PJ, Bernard S, Sarradin P, et al. IMPY, a potential beta-amyloid imaging probe for detection of prion deposits in scrapie-infected mice. Nucl Med Biol 2008;35(2):197–201.

101. Lin KS, Debnath ML, Mathis CA, et al. Synthesis and beta-amyloid binding properties of rhenium 2-phenylbenzothiazoles. Bioorg Med Chem Lett 2009;19(8):2258–62.

102. Qu W, Kung MP, Hou C, et al. Novel styrylpyridines as probes for SPECT imaging of amyloid plaques. J Med Chem 2007;50(9):2157–65.

103. Qu W, Kung MP, Hou C, et al. Radioiodinated aza-diphenylacetylenes as potential SPECT imaging agents for beta-amyloid plaque detection. Bioorg Med Chem Lett 2007;17(13):3581–4.

104. Serdons K, Verduyckt T, Cleynhens J, et al. Synthesis and evaluation of a (99m)Tc-BAT-phenyl-benzothiazole conjugate as a potential in vivo tracer for visualization of amyloid beta. Bioorg Med Chem Lett 2007;17(22):6086–90.

105. Price JC, Klunk WE, Lopresti BJ, et al. Kinetic modeling of amyloid binding in humans using PET imaging and Pittsburgh Compound-B. J Cereb Blood Flow Metab 2005;25(11):1528–47.

106. Lockhart A, Ye L, Judd DB, et al. Evidence for the presence of three distinct binding sites for the thio-flavin T class of Alzheimer's disease PET imaging agents on beta-amyloid peptide fibrils. J Biol Chem 2005;280(9):7677–84.

107. Ye L, Morgenstern JL, Gee AD, et al. Delineation of positron emission tomography imaging agent binding sites on beta-amyloid peptide fibrils. J Biol Chem 2005;280(25):23599–604.

108. Klunk WE, Lopresti BJ, Ikonomovic MD, et al. Binding of the positron emission tomography tracer Pittsburgh compound-B reflects the amount of amyloid-beta in Alzheimer's disease brain but not in transgenic mouse brain. J Neurosci 2005; 25(46):10598–606.

109. Maeda J, Ji B, Irie T, et al. Longitudinal, quantitative assessment of amyloid, neuroinflammation, and anti-amyloid treatment in a living mouse model of Alzheimer's disease enabled by positron emission tomography. J Neurosci 2007; 27(41):10957–68.

110. Fodero-Tavoletti MT, Rowe CC, McLean CA, et al. Characterization of PiB binding to white matter in Alzheimer disease and other dementias. J Nucl Med 2009;50(2):198–204.

111. LeVine H 3rd. Quantification of beta-sheet amyloid fibril structures with thioflavin T. Meth Enzymol 1999;309:274–84.

112. Lockhart A, Lamb JR, Osredkar T, et al. PIB is a non-specific imaging marker of amyloid-beta (Abeta) peptide-related cerebral amyloidosis. Brain 2007;130(Pt 10):2607–15.

113. Fodero-Tavoletti MT, Smith DP, McLean CA, et al. In vitro characterization of Pittsburgh compound-B binding to Lewy bodies. J Neurosci 2007;27(39):10365–71.

114. Ye L, Velasco A, Fraser G, et al. In vitro high affinity alpha-synuclein binding sites for the amyloid imaging agent PIB are not matched by binding to Lewy bodies in postmortem human brain. J Neurochem 2008;105(4):1428–37.

115. Ikonomovic MD, Klunk WE, Abrahamson EE, et al. Post-mortem correlates of in vivo PiB-PET amyloid imaging in a typical case of Alzheimer's disease. Brain 2008;131(Pt 6):1630–45.

116. Trojanowski JQ. Emerging Alzheimer's disease therapies: focusing on the future. Neurobiol Aging 2002;23(6):985–90.

117. Kung MP, Hou C, Zhuang ZP, et al. Binding of two potential imaging agents targeting amyloid plaques in postmortem brain tissues of patients with Alzheimer's disease. Brain Res 2004;1025(1–2):98–105.

118. Okamura N, Suemoto T, Shimadzu H, et al. Styryl-benzoxazole derivatives for in vivo imaging of amyloid plaques in the brain. J Neurosci 2004; 24(10):2535–41.

119. Kudo Y. Development of amyloid imaging PET probes for an early diagnosis of Alzheimer's disease. Minim Invasive Ther Allied Technol 2006; 15(4):209–13.

120. Fodero-Tavoletti MT, Mulligan RS, Okamura N, et al. In vitro characterisation of BF227 binding to alpha-synuclein/Lewy bodies. Eur J Pharmacol 2009;617:54–8.

121. Okamura N, Furumoto S, Furukawa K, et al. PET imaging of brain Amyloid deposits using BF-227 and its derivative [abstract]. Alzheimers Dement 2008;4(Suppl 1):T383.

122. Johnson AE, Jeppsson F, Sandell J, et al. AZD2184: a radioligand for sensitive detection of beta-amyloid deposits. J Neurochem 2009;108(5): 1177–86.

123. Agdeppa ED, Kepe V, Shoghi-Jadid K, et al. In vivo and in vitro labeling of plaques and tangles in the brain of an Alzheimer's disease patient: a case study. J Nucl Med 2001;42(Suppl 1):65P.

124. Agdeppa ED, Kepe V, Liu J, et al. Binding characteristics of radiofluorinated 6-dialkylamino-2-naphthylethylidene derivatives as positron emission tomography imaging probes for beta-amyloid plaques in Alzheimer's disease. J Neurosci 2001; 21(24):RC189.

125. Barrio JR, Huang SC, Cole G, et al. PET imaging of tangles and plaques in Alzheimer disease with a highly hydrophobic probe. J Labelled Compd Radiopharm 1999;42:S194–5.

126. Bresjanac M, Smid LM, Vovko TD, et al. Molecular-imaging probe 2-(1-[6-[(2-fluoroethyl)(methyl) amino]-2-naphthyl]ethylidene) malononitrile labels prion plaques in vitro. J Neurosci 2003;23(22): 8029–33.

127. Small GW, Agdeppa ED, Kepe V, et al. In vivo brain imaging of tangle burden in humans. J Mol Neurosci 2002;19(3):323–7.

128. Small GW, Kepe V, Ercoli LM, et al. PET of brain amyloid and tau in mild cognitive impairment. N Engl J Med 2006;355(25):2652–63.

129. Noda A, Murakami Y, Nishiyama S, et al. Amyloid imaging in aged and young macaques with [^{11}C]PIB and [^{18}F]FDDNP. Synapse 2008;62(6): 472–5.

130. Tolboom N, Yaqub M, van der Flier WM, et al. Detection of Alzheimer pathology in vivo using both ^{11}C-PIB and ^{18}F-FDDNP PET. J Nucl Med 2009;50(2):191–7.

131. Shih WJ, Markesbery WR, Clark DB, et al. Iodine-123 HIPDM brain imaging findings in subacute spongiform encephalopathy (Creutzfeldt-Jakob disease). J Nucl Med 1987;28(9):1484–7.

132. Thompson PW, Ye L, Morgenstern JL, et al. Interaction of the amyloid imaging tracer FDDNP with hallmark Alzheimer's disease pathologies. J Neurochem 2009;109(2):623–30.

133. Zhang W, Oya S, Kung MP, et al. F-18 stilbenes as PET imaging agents for detecting beta-amyloid plaques in the brain. J Med Chem 2005;48(19): 5980–8.

134. Zhang W, Oya S, Kung MP, et al. F-18 Polyethyleneglycol stilbenes as PET imaging agents targeting Abeta aggregates in the brain. Nucl Med Biol 2005;32(8):799–809.

135. Doraiswamy PM, Farmer M, Holub R, et al. Relationship between regional amyloid levels and cognitive performance in healthy controls, MCI subjects, and patients with Alzheimer's: Phase II results from a florpiramine F18 PET imaging study. Alzheimers Dement 2009; 5(4 Suppl 1):P77.

136. Sperling R, Johnson K, Pontecorvo MJ, et al. PET imaging of beta-amyloid with florpiramine F18 (18F-AV-45): Preliminary results from a phase II study of cognitively normal elderly subjects, individuals with mild cognitive impairment, and patients with a clinical diagnosis of Alzheimer's disease [abstract]. Alzheimers Dement 2009; 5(4 Suppl 1):P197.

137. Serdons K, Verduyckt T, Vanderghinste D, et al. Synthesis of ^{18}F-labelled 2-(4'-fluorophenyl)-1,3-benzothiazole and evaluation as amyloid imaging agent in comparison with [11C]PIB. Bioorg Med Chem Lett 2009;19(3):602–5.

138. Mathis CA, Ikonomovic MD, Mason NS, et al. Pharmacologic and pharmacokinetic equivalence studies of GE-067 to PiB [abstract]. Alzheimers Dement 2009;5(4 Suppl 1):P262.

139. Van Laere K, Vanderberghe R, Ivaniou A, et al. Correlation between 18F-GE-067 and 11C-PIB uptake in Alzheimer's disease and MCI [abstract]. Alzheimers Dement 2009;5(4 Suppl 1):P263.

140. Sundgren-Andersson AK, Svensson SPS, Swahn BM, et al. AZD4694: fluorinated positron emission tomography (PET) radioligand for detection of beta-amyloid deposits [abstract]. Alzheimers Dement 2009;5(4 Suppl 1):P267–8.

141. Rowe CC, Ng S, Ackermann U, et al. Imaging beta-amyloid burden in aging and dementia. Neurology 2007;68(20):1718–25.

142. Forsberg A, Engler H, Almkvist O, et al. PET imaging of amyloid deposition in patients with mild cognitive impairment. Neurobiol Aging 2008; 29(10):1456–65.

143. Mintun MA, Larossa GN, Sheline YI, et al. [^{11}C]PIB in a nondemented population: potential antecedent marker of Alzheimer disease. Neurology 2006; 67(3):446–52.

144. Gomperts SN, Rentz DM, Moran E, et al. Imaging amyloid deposition in Lewy body diseases. Neurology 2008;71(12):903–10.

145. Maetzler W, Liepelt I, Reimold M, et al. Cortical PIB binding in Lewy body disease is associated with

Alzheimer-like characteristics. Neurobiol Dis 2009; 34(1):107–12.

146. Lopresti BJ, Klunk WE, Mathis CA, et al. Simplified quantification of Pittsburgh Compound B amyloid imaging PET studies: a comparative analysis. J Nucl Med 2005;46(12):1959–72.

147. Joachim CL, Morris JH, Selkoe DJ. Diffuse senile plaques occur commonly in the cerebellum in Alzheimer's disease. Am J Pathol 1989;135(2):309–19.

148. Klunk WE, Price JC, Mathis CA, et al. Amyloid deposition begins in the striatum of presenilin-1 mutation carriers from two unrelated pedigrees. J Neurosci 2007;27(23):6174–84.

149. Koivunen J, Verkkoniemi A, Aalto S, et al. PET amyloid ligand [^{11}C]PIB uptake shows predominantly striatal increase in variant Alzheimer's disease. Brain 2008;131(Pt 7):1845–53.

150. Boxer AL, Rabinovici GD, Kepe V, et al. Amyloid imaging in distinguishing atypical prion disease from Alzheimer disease. Neurology 2007;69(3): 283–90.

151. Villemagne VL, McLean CA, Reardon K, et al. ^{11}C-PiB PET studies in typical sporadic Creutzfeldt-Jakob disease. J Neurol Neurosurg Psychiatr 2009; 66:1537–44.

152. Johansson A, Savitcheva I, Forsberg A, et al. [(11)C]-PIB imaging in patients with Parkinson's disease: preliminary results. Parkinsonism Relat Disord 2008;14(4):345–7.

153. Edison P, Rowe CC, Rinne JO, et al. Amyloid load in Parkinson's disease dementia and Lewy body dementia measured with [^{11}C]PIB positron emission tomography. J Neurol Neurosurg Psychiatr 2008;79(12):1331–8.

154. Maetzler W, Reimold M, Liepelt I, et al. [^{11}C]PIB binding in Parkinson's disease dementia. Neuroimage 2008;39(3):1027–33.

155. Ng SY, Villemagne VL, Masters CL, et al. Evaluating atypical dementia syndromes using positron emission tomography with carbon 11 labeled Pittsburgh Compound B. Arch Neurol 2007;64(8):1140–4.

156. Braak H, Braak E. Frequency of stages of Alzheimer-related lesions in different age categories. Neurobiol Aging 1997;18(4):351–7.

157. Thal DR, Rub U, Orantes M, et al. Phases of A beta-deposition in the human brain and its relevance for the development of AD. Neurology 2002;58:1791–800.

158. Bacskai BJ, Frosch MP, Freeman SH, et al. Molecular imaging with Pittsburgh Compound B confirmed at autopsy: a case report. Arch Neurol 2007;64(3):431–4.

159. Arnold SE, Han LY, Clark CM, et al. Quantitative neurohistological features of frontotemporal degeneration. Neurobiol Aging 2000;21(6):913–9.

160. Leinonen V, Alafuzoff I, Aalto S, et al. Assessment of beta-amyloid in a frontal cortical brain biopsy specimen and by positron emission tomography with carbon 11-labeled Pittsburgh Compound B. Arch Neurol 2008;65(10):1304–9.

161. Johnson KA, Gregas M, Becker JA, et al. Imaging of amyloid burden and distribution in cerebral amyloid angiopathy. Ann Neurol 2007; 62(3):229–34.

162. Drzezga A, Grimmer T, Henriksen G, et al. Imaging of amyloid plaques and cerebral glucose metabolism in semantic dementia and Alzheimer's disease. Neuroimage 2008;39(2):619–33.

163. Engler H, Santillo AF, Wang SX, et al. In vivo amyloid imaging with PET in frontotemporal dementia. Eur J Nucl Med Mol Imaging 2008; 35(1):100–6.

164. Rabinovici GD, Furst AJ, O'Neil JP, et al. ^{11}C-PIB PET imaging in Alzheimer disease and frontotemporal lobar degeneration. Neurology 2007;68(15): 1205–12.

165. Rabinovici GD, Jagust WJ, Furst AJ, et al. Abeta amyloid and glucose metabolism in three variants of primary progressive aphasia. Ann Neurol 2008; 64(4):388–401.

166. Morris JC, Storandt M, Miller JP, et al. Mild cognitive impairment represents early-stage Alzheimer disease. Arch Neurol 2001;58(3):397–405.

167. Kemppainen NM, Aalto S, Wilson IA, et al. PET amyloid ligand [^{11}C]PIB uptake is increased in mild cognitive impairment. Neurology 2007; 68(19):1603–6.

168. Pike KE, Savage G, Villemagne VL, et al. Beta-amyloid imaging and memory in non-demented individuals: evidence for preclinical Alzheimer's disease. Brain 2007;130(Pt 11):2837–44.

169. Villemagne VL, Pike KE, Darby D, et al. Abeta deposits in older non-demented individuals with cognitive decline are indicative of preclinical Alzheimer's disease. Neuropsychologia 2008;46(6): 1688–97.

170. Aizenstein HJ, Nebes RD, Saxton JA, et al. Frequent amyloid deposition without significant cognitive impairment among the elderly. Arch Neurol 2008;65(11):1509–17.

171. Davies L, Wolska B, Hilbich C, et al. A4 amyloid protein deposition and the diagnosis of Alzheimer's disease: prevalence in aged brains determined by immunocytochemistry compared with conventional neuropathologic techniques. Neurology 1988; 38(11):1688–93.

172. Forman MS, Mufson EJ, Leurgans S, et al. Cortical biochemistry in MCI and Alzheimer disease: lack of correlation with clinical diagnosis. Neurology 2007; 68(10):757–63.

173. Morris JC, Price AL. Pathologic correlates of nondemented aging, mild cognitive impairment, and early-stage Alzheimer's disease. J Mol Neurosci 2001;17(2):101–18.

174. Hof PR, Glannakopoulos P, Bouras C. The neuro-pathological changes associated with normal brain aging. Histol Histopathol 1996; 11(4):1075–88.

175. Thal DR, Del Tredici K, Braak H. Neurodegeneration in normal brain aging and disease. Sci Aging Knowledge Environ 2004;2004(23):pe26.

176. Backman L, Jones S, Berger AK, et al. Cognitive impairment in preclinical Alzheimer's disease: a meta-analysis. Neuropsychology 2005;19(4): 520–31.

177. Small BJ, Gagnon E, Robinson B. Early identification of cognitive deficits: preclinical Alzheimer's disease and mild cognitive impairment. Geriatrics 2007;62(4):19–23.

178. Price JL, Morris JC. Tangles and plaques in nondemented aging and "preclinical" Alzheimer's disease. Ann Neurol 1999;45(3):358–68.

179. Nordberg A. Amyloid imaging in Alzheimer's disease. Curr Opin Neurol 2007;20(4):398–402.

180. Fagan AM, Roe CM, Xiong C, et al. Cerebrospinal fluid tau/beta-amyloid(42) ratio as a prediction of cognitive decline in nondemented older adults. Arch Neurol 2007;64(3):343–9.

181. Fagan AM, Mintun MA, Mach RH, et al. Inverse relation between in vivo amyloid imaging load and cerebrospinal fluid Abeta(42) in humans. Ann Neurol 2006;59(3):512–9.

182. Koivunen J, Pirttila T, Kemppainen N, et al. PET amyloid ligand [C]PIB uptake and cerebrospinal fluid beta-amyloid in mild cognitive impairment. Dement Geriatr Cogn Disord 2008;26(4):378–83.

183. Archer HA, Edison P, Brooks DJ, et al. Amyloid load and cerebral atrophy in Alzheimer's disease: an ^{11}C-PIB positron emission tomography study. Ann Neurol 2006;60(1):145–7.

184. Jack CR Jr, Lowe VJ, Senjem ML, et al. [11]C PiB and structural MRI provide complementary information in imaging of Alzheimer's disease and amnestic mild cognitive impairment. Brain 2008;131(Pt 3): 665–80.

185. Frisoni GB, Lorenzi M, Caroli A, et al. In vivo mapping of amyloid toxicity in Alzheimer disease. Neurology 2009;72(17):1504–11.

186. Mormino EC, Kluth JT, Madison CM, et al. Episodic memory loss is related to hippocampal-mediated beta-amyloid deposition in elderly subjects. Brain 2009;132(Pt 5):1310–23.

187. Bennett DA, Schneider JA, Arvanitakis Z, et al. Neuropathology of older persons without cognitive impairment from two community-based studies. Neurology 2006;66(12):1837–44.

188. Edison P, Archer HA, Hinz R, et al. Amyloid, hypometabolism, and cognition in Alzheimer disease: an [11C]PIB and [18F]FDG PET study. Neurology 2007;68(7):501–8.

189. Li Y, Rinne JO, Mosconi L, et al. Regional analysis of FDG and PIB-PET images in normal aging, mild cognitive impairment, and Alzheimer's disease. Eur J Nucl Med Mol Imaging 2008;35:2169–89.

190. Ng S, Villemagne VL, Berlangieri S, et al. Visual assessment versus quantitative assessment of ^{11}C-PIB PET and ^{18}F-FDG PET for detection of Alzheimer's disease. J Nucl Med 2007;48(4):547–52.

191. Strittmatter WJ, Saunders AM, Schmechel D, et al. Apolipoprotein E: high-avidity binding to beta-amyloid and increased frequency of type 4 allele in late-onset familial Alzheimer disease. Proc Natl Acad Sci U S A 1993;90(5):1977–81.

192. Martins IJ, Hone E, Foster JK, et al. Apolipoprotein E, cholesterol metabolism, diabetes, and the convergence of risk factors for Alzheimer's disease and cardiovascular disease. Mol Psychiatry 2006; 11(8):721–36.

193. Ritchie K, Dupuy AM. The current status of apo E4 as a risk factor for Alzheimer's disease: an epidemiological perspective. Int J Geriatr Psychiatry 1999;14(9):695–700.

194. Reiman EM, Chen K, Liu X, et al. Fibrillar amyloid-beta burden in cognitively normal people at 3 levels of genetic risk for Alzheimer's disease. Proc Natl Acad Sci U S A 2009;106(16):6820–5.

195. Villemagne VL, Ataka S, Brooks W, et al. Pattern of Abeta deposition in familial Alzheimer's disease is irrespective of mutation type or cognitive status [abstract]. J Nucl Med 2008;49(Suppl 1):216P.

196. Wolk DA, Price JC, Saxton JA, et al. Amyloid imaging in mild cognitive impairment subtypes. Ann Neurol 2009;65(5):557–68.

197. Okello A, Koivunen J, Edison P, et al. Conversion of amyloid positive and negative MCI to AD over 3 years. An ^{11}C-PIB PET study. Neurology 2009;73: 754–60.

198. Buckner RL, Snyder AZ, Shannon BJ, et al. Molecular, structural, and functional characterization of Alzheimer's disease: evidence for a relationship between default activity, amyloid, and memory. J Neurosci 2005;25(34):7709–17.

199. Buckner RL, Andrews-Hanna JR, Schacter DL. The brain's default network: anatomy, function, and relevance to disease. Ann N Y Acad Sci 2008; 1124:1–38.

200. Wermke M, Sorg C, Wohlschlager AM, et al. A new integrative model of cerebral activation, deactivation and default mode function in Alzheimer's disease. Eur J Nucl Med Mol Imaging 2008; 35(Suppl 1):S12–24.

201. Engler H, Forsberg A, Almkvist O, et al. Two-year follow-up of amyloid deposition in patients with Alzheimer's disease. Brain 2006;129(Pt 11):2856–66.

202. Jack CR Jr, Lowe VJ, Weigand SD, et al. Serial PIB and MRI in normal, mild cognitive impairment and Alzheimer's disease: implications for sequence of

pathological events in Alzheimer's disease. Brain 2009;132(Pt 5):1355–65.

203. Ellis KA, Bush AI, Darby D, et al. The Australian Imaging, Biomarkers and Lifestyle (AIBL) study of aging: methodology and baseline characteristics of 1112 individuals recruited for a longitudinal study of Alzheimer's disease. Int Psychogeriatr 2009;21(4):672–87.

204. Mueller SG, Weiner MW, Thal LJ, et al. The Alzheimer's disease neuroimaging initiative. Neuroimaging Clin N Am 2005;15(4):869–77, xi-xii.

205. Eckert A, Keil U, Marques CA, et al. Mitochondrial dysfunction, apoptotic cell death, and Alzheimer's disease. Biochem Pharmacol 2003; 66(8):1627–34.

206. Leuner K, Hauptmann S, Abdel-Kader R, et al. Mitochondrial dysfunction: the first domino in brain aging and Alzheimer's disease? Antioxid Redox Signal 2007;9(10):1659–75.

207. Suo Z, Wu M, Citron BA, et al. Abnormality of G-protein-coupled receptor kinases at prodromal and early stages of Alzheimer's disease: an association with early beta-amyloid accumulation. J Neurosci 2004;24(13):3444–52.

208. Resende R, Pereira C, Agostinho P, et al. Susceptibility of hippocampal neurons to Abeta peptide toxicity is associated with perturbation of Ca^{2+} homeostasis. Brain Res 2007;1143:11–21.

209. Roder S, Danober L, Pozza MF, et al. Electrophysiological studies on the hippocampus and prefrontal cortex assessing the effects of amyloidosis in amyloid precursor protein 23 transgenic mice. Neuroscience 2003;120(3):705–20.

210. Capetillo-Zarate E, Staufenbiel M, Abramowski D, et al. Selective vulnerability of different types of commissural neurons for amyloid beta-protein-induced neurodegeneration in APP23 mice correlates with dendritic tree morphology. Brain 2006; 129(Pt 11):2992–3005.

211. Kemppainen NM, Aalto S, Karrasch M, et al. Cognitive reserve hypothesis: Pittsburgh Compound B and fluorodeoxyglucose positron emission tomography in relation to education in mild Alzheimer's disease. Ann Neurol 2008;63(1):112–8.

212. Mortimer JA. Brain reserve and the clinical expression of Alzheimer's disease. Geriatrics 1997; 52(Suppl 2):S50–3.

213. Stern Y. What is cognitive reserve? Theory and research application of the reserve concept. J Int Neuropsychol Soc 2002;8(3):448–60.

214. Roe CM, Mintun MA, D'Angelo G, et al. Alzheimer disease and cognitive reserve: variation of education effect with carbon 11-labeled Pittsburgh Compound B uptake. Arch Neurol 2008;65(11): 1467–71.

215. Deshpande A, Mina E, Glabe C, et al. Different conformations of amyloid beta induce neurotoxicity

by distinct mechanisms in human cortical neurons. J Neurosci 2006;26(22):6011–8.

216. Walker LC, Rosen RF, Levine H 3rd. Diversity of Abeta deposits in the aged brain: a window on molecular heterogeneity? Rom J Morphol Embryol 2008;49(1):5–11.

217. Levine H 3rd, Walker LC. Molecular polymorphism of Abeta in Alzheimer's disease. Neurobiol Aging 2010;31(4):542–8.

218. Rosen RF, Walker LC, Levine H 3rd. PIB binding in aged primate brain: Enrichment of high-affinity sites in humans with Alzheimer's disease. Neurobiol Aging 2010;31(4):542–8.

219. Clark CM, Davatzikos C, Borthakur A, et al. Biomarkers for early detection of Alzheimer pathology. Neurosignals 2008;16(1):11–8.

220. Shaw LM, Korecka M, Clark CM, et al. Biomarkers of neurodegeneration for diagnosis and monitoring therapeutics. Nat Rev Drug Discov 2007;6(4):295–303.

221. Hoglund K, Hansson O, Buchhave P, et al. Prediction of Alzheimer's disease using a cerebrospinal fluid pattern of C-terminally truncated beta-amyloid peptides. Neurodegener Dis 2008; 5(5):268–76.

222. Hansson O, Zetterberg H, Buchhave P, et al. Prediction of Alzheimer's disease using the CSF Abeta42/Abeta40 ratio in patients with mild cognitive impairment. Dement Geriatr Cogn Disord 2007;23(5):316–20.

223. Hansson O, Zetterberg H, Buchhave P, et al. Association between CSF biomarkers and incipient Alzheimer's disease in patients with mild cognitive impairment: a follow-up study. Lancet Neurol 2006;5(3):228–34.

224. Thompson PM, Hayashi KM, de Zubicaray G, et al. Dynamics of gray matter loss in Alzheimer's disease. J Neurosci 2003;23(3):994–1005.

225. Small GW. Diagnostic issues in dementia: neuroimaging as a surrogate marker of disease. J Geriatr Psychiatry Neurol 2006;19(3):180–5.

226. de Leon MJ, DeSanti S, Zinkowski R, et al. MRI and CSF studies in the early diagnosis of Alzheimer's disease. J Intern Med 2004;256(3):205–23.

227. Modrego PJ. Predictors of conversion to dementia of probable Alzheimer type in patients with mild cognitive impairment. Curr Alzheimer Res 2006; 3(2):161–70.

228. Smith EE, Egorova S, Blacker D, et al. Magnetic resonance imaging white matter hyperintensities and brain volume in the prediction of mild cognitive impairment and dementia. Arch Neurol 2008;65(1): 94–100.

229. van de Pol LA, van der Flier WM, Korf ES, et al. Baseline predictors of rates of hippocampal atrophy in mild cognitive impairment. Neurology 2007;69(15):1491–7.

230. Stoub TR, Bulgakova M, Leurgans S, et al. MRI predictors of risk of incident Alzheimer disease: a longitudinal study. Neurology 2005;64(9):1520–4.

231. Spulber G, Niskanen E, Macdonald S, et al. Whole brain atrophy rate predicts progression from MCI to Alzheimer's disease. Neurobiol Aging 2008. DOI:10.1016/j.neurobiolaging.2008.08.018.

232. Jack CR Jr, Shiung MM, Weigand SD, et al. Brain atrophy rates predict subsequent clinical conversion in normal elderly and amnestic MCI. Neurology 2005;65(8):1227–31.

233. Silverman DH, Cummings JL, Small G, et al. Added clinical benefit of incorporating 2-deoxy-2-[^{18}F]fluoro-D-glucose with positron emission tomography into the clinical evaluation of patients with cognitive impairment. Mol Imaging Biol 2002;4(4):283–9.

234. Small GW, Mazziotta JC, Collins MT, et al. Apolipoprotein E type 4 allele and cerebral glucose metabolism in relatives at risk for familial Alzheimer disease. JAMA 1995;273(12):942–7.

235. Silverman DH, Small GW, Chang CY, et al. Positron emission tomography in evaluation of dementia: regional brain metabolism and long-term outcome. JAMA 2001;286(17):2120–7.

236. Silverman DH, Chang CY, Cummings JL, et al. Prognostic value of regional brain metabolism in evaluation of dementia. J Nucl Med 1999;40(Suppl 1):71P.

237. Chang CY, Silverman DH. Accuracy of early diagnosis and its impact on the management and course of Alzheimer's disease. Expert Rev Mol Diagn 2004;4:63–9.

238. Silverman DH, Gambhir SS, Huang HW, et al. Evaluating early dementia with and without assessment of regional cerebral metabolism by PET: a comparison of predicted costs and benefits. J Nucl Med 2002;43(2):253–66.

239. Drzezga A, Lautenschlager N, Siebner H, et al. Cerebral metabolic changes accompanying conversion of mild cognitive impairment into Alzheimer's disease: a PET follow-up study. Eur J Nucl Med Mol Imaging 2003;30(8):1104–13.

240. Drzezga A, Grimmer T, Riemenschneider M, et al. Prediction of individual clinical outcome in MCI by means of genetic assessment and (18)F-FDG PET. J Nucl Med 2005;46(10):1625–32.

241. Frank RA, Galasko D, Hampel H, et al. Biological markers for therapeutic trials in Alzheimer's disease. Proceedings of the biological markers working group; NIA initiative on neuroimaging in Alzheimer's disease. Neurobiol Aging 2003;24(4):521–36.

242. Zetterberg H, Blennow K. Plasma Abeta in Alzheimer's disease—up or down? Lancet Neurol 2006;5(8):638–9.

243. Raymond SB, Skoch J, Hills ID, et al. Smart optical probes for near-infrared fluorescence imaging of Alzheimer's disease pathology. Eur J Nucl Med Mol Imaging 2008;35(Suppl 1):S93–8.

244. Hintersteiner M, Enz A, Frey P, et al. In vivo detection of amyloid-beta deposits by near-infrared imaging using an oxazine-derivative probe. Nat Biotechnol 2005;23(5):577–83.

^{18}F-Fluorodeoxyglucose PET in the Evaluation of Parkinson Disease

Kathleen L. Poston, MD, MS[a], David Eidelberg, MD[b,c],*

KEYWORDS

- Positron emission tomography • Parkinsonism
- Movement disorders • Differential diagnosis
- Brain metabolism • Biomarkers • Treatment response

Parkinson disease (PD) is the second most common age-related neurodegenerative disorder, affecting 1 to 2 million individuals in North America. Given that the incidence of PD increases with age, the number of PD patients is estimated to triple in the next 50 years as the average age of the population increases.[1] Classically, PD is defined by motor features of bradykinesia (slow movement), rest tremor, muscle rigidity, and gait abnormalities. However, nonmotor features, including cognitive decline, dementia, and depression, can significantly contribute to patient disability and can even increase mortality.[2,3] Diagnosis is typically made solely on clinical findings and can be challenging, particularly early in the disease course. Even among specialists, diagnosis at disease onset can be elusive, as the clinical symptoms in early PD overlap with several "look-alike" disorders.[4] Conventional anatomic imaging techniques, such as magnetic resonance (MR) imaging and computed tomography, are generally not helpful in diagnosing PD, particularly in early patients, nor are they helpful in monitoring changes in disease over time. More accurate clinical diagnosis requires at least 2 years of clinical follow-up by a movement disorders specialist with expertise in rarer causes of parkinsonism, such as progressive supranuclear palsy (PSP) and multiple system atrophy (MSA).[4] These more aggressive and less treatable syndromes are the most common atypical forms of parkinsonism misdiagnosed as PD[5]; therefore accurate diagnosis is critical for patient counseling and treatment decisions.

Current research in neurodegenerative diseases has centered on the development of biomarkers to aid clinicians and researchers in making earlier, more accurate diagnoses, specifically in PD and other atypical parkinsonian disorders.[6] In addition, biomarkers for the objective assessment of disease progression and response to treatment are critical for researching new therapies for these progressive, incurable diseases. Indeed, such biomarkers are vital to the development of potentially neuromodulatory medical and surgical treatments for PD, including cell-based approaches[7] and gene transfer therapy.[8,9]

Functional imaging with PET has the potential to fulfill the need for such biomarkers by providing objective, quantifiable, and stable markers for the diagnosis of parkinsonian syndromes, and for the assessment of the progression and response to

This work was supported by NIH NINDS R01 NS 035069, R01 NS 37564, P50 NS 38370, and the General Clinical Research Center of The Feinstein Institute for Medical Research (M01 RR018535).

^a Department of Neurology and Neurological Sciences, Stanford University Medical Center, 300 Pasteur Drive, Room A343, Stanford, CA 94305-5235, USA

^b Center for Neurosciences, The Feinstein Institute for Medical Research, North Shore-Long Island Jewish Health System, 350 Community Drive, Manhasset, NY 11030, USA

^c Departments of Neurology and Medicine, North Shore University Hospital, 300 Community Drive, Manhasset, NY, USA

* Corresponding author. Center for Neurosciences, The Feinstein Institute for Medical Research, North Shore-Long Island Jewish Health System, 350 Community Drive, Manhasset, NY 11030.

E-mail address: david1@nshs.edu

PET Clin 5 (2010) 55–64

doi:10.1016/j.cpet.2009.12.004

treatment of these disorders. Over a decade ago it was first recognized that regional differences in glucose metabolism measured with ^{18}F-fluoro-deoxyglucose (FDG) PET could be used to distinguish between different forms of parkinsonism.[10] However, broad application of metabolic imaging in these neurodegenerative diseases has been limited because of the substantial variability in brain activity between subjects and difficulty analyzing large datasets. A relatively novel approach that aims to overcome these limitations is a spatial covariance method based on principal components analysis (PCA).[11] This method, termed the scaled subprofile model (SSM), has been applied to FDG PET scans to identify disease-specific metabolic patterns in patients with various neurodegenerative disorders.[12,13] Indeed, spatial covariance mapping has been used with FDG PET to identify abnormal metabolic patterns (ie, large-scale brain networks) associated with a variety of neurodegenerative diseases, including PD, MSA, PSP, Alzheimer disease,[14] and Huntington disease.[15]

In this review, the authors describe current applications of FDG PET with pattern analysis to the characterization of parkinsonian disorders. The article focuses on the use of this approach in aiding clinical diagnosis, in monitoring disease progression, and in studying novel treatments for PD and related disorders.

METABOLIC NETWORKS IN PARKINSONISM
The PD-Related Motor Pattern

The cardinal motor abnormalities of PD have been attributed not only to dysfunction within the basal ganglia but also to broader functional abnormalities involving the corticostriato-pallido-thalamo-cortical (CSPTC) and related pathways.[16] Therefore, it is not surprising that the abnormal spatial covariance pattern consistently identified in PD patients involves metabolic changes at key nodes of these circuits.[17–19] This PD-related metabolic pattern (PDRP) is characterized by increased pallidothalamic and pontine metabolic activity associated with relative reductions in premotor cortex, supplementary motor area, and in parietal association areas (**Fig. 1**, *left*). Indeed, similar PDRP topographies have been detected in 7 independent patient populations using a variety of resting-state imaging techniques.[12]

By forward application of networks into individual cases, disease-related spatial patterns can be quantified prospectively in single scans.[13] Indeed, PDRP subject scores, measuring pattern expression in individual subjects, have been found to be highly reproducible with stable network activity recorded over hours to weeks.[20] In PD patients, pattern expression has been found to correlate with validated clinical markers of disease severity, such as standardized motor rating scales and symptom duration.[21,22] However, unlike

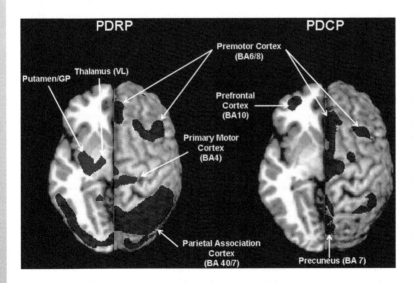

Fig. 1. Parkinson disease (PD)-related spatial covariance patterns. (*Left*) PD motor-related spatial covariance pattern (PDRP[20]) characterized by pallidothalamic, pontine, and motor cortical hypermetabolism, associated with relative metabolic reductions in the lateral premotor and posterior parietal areas. (*Right*) PD cognition-related spatial covariance pattern (PDCP[28]) characterized by hypometabolism of prefrontal cortex, rostral supplementary motor area, and superior parietal regions. Relative metabolic increases are displayed in red; relative metabolic decreases are displayed in blue. Both patterns were overlaid on a standard MR imaging brain template. The left hemisphere was cut in the transverse plane at z = −5 mm. The right hemisphere was displayed as a surface projection on the same brain template. (*Reprinted from* Hirano S, Asanuma K, Ma Y, et al. Dissociation of metabolic and neurovascular responses to levodopa in the treatment of Parkinson's disease. J Neurosci 2008;28:4203, copyright 2008 The Society for Neuroscience; with permission.)

clinical ratings, PDRP scores are fully objective and unbiased by inter-rater variability. Also, current PD rating scales, such as the Unified Parkinson's Disease Rating Scale (UPDRS),[23] are relatively more sensitive for detecting changes in certain motor aspects of disease, such as worsening tremor or bradykinesia. However, these clinical scales are less sensitive to changes in other PD symptoms, such as freezing of gait and falls, and may therefore fail to capture total motor progression in many patients. The PDRP, however, is generated without a priori assumptions regarding patient symptomatology and is present regardless of patient phenotype.[24,25] Although the correlations between the motor UPDRS and PDRP activity are significant and consistent across populations, the overall effect is modest, with 40% to 50% variability in common for the 2 measures.[13] Indeed, rather than being a biomarker for specific clinical manifestations of PD, PDRP expression likely reflects overall abnormalities in motor circuitry associated with this neurodegenerative disease.

The PD-Related Cognitive Pattern

Cognitive disturbances, including mild cognitive impairment (MCI) and PD dementia (PDD), are among the most concerning nonmotor symptoms in PD and are present in more than 80% of patients with 15 years of disease duration.[2] Indeed, dementia is associated with a doubling of mortality risk in older patients with PD.[26] Earlier in the course of the disease, a wide variety of more subtle cognitive changes occur, the most prominent being deficits in executive function, followed by visuospatial and working memory deficits.[27] Clinically, these cognitive changes are nonresponsive to therapies aimed at treating PD motor symptoms and develop later in the disease course. Therefore, PD-associated cognitive symptoms are generally attributed to a separate set of regional changes than the motor symptoms.[28,29]

FDG PET with spatial covariance analysis has also been used to study the cognitive changes associated with PD. A voxel-based spatial covariance approach has been used to identify a specific PDRP associated with cognitive dysfunction in nondemented patients.[28] This PD-related cognitive pattern (PDCP) is characterized by metabolic reductions in the medial, frontal, and parietal association regions with relative increases in the cerebellar vermis and dentate nuclei (see Fig. 1, *right*). This pattern is distinct from the PDRP, and its expression has been shown to correlate with performance on neuropsychological tests of executive functioning and memory. Indeed, PDCP expression was found to increase stepwise in PD patients categorized clinically by the degree of cognitive impairment on a psychometric battery.[29,30] Similar to the PDRP, PDCP expression is highly reproducible in individual patients.[20] Although both PDRP and PDCP expression increase with disease duration, PDCP increases at a slower rate, reflecting the relatively later development of neurodegenerative changes in the cerebral cortex.[30] Indeed, the findings suggest that the PDCP metabolic network can be used as a specific biomarker for the evaluation of cognitive dysfunction in PD patients.

METABOLIC PATTERNS IN ATYPICAL PARKINSONIAN SYNDROMES

Atypical parkinsonian syndromes (APS) share many clinical symptoms seen in classical PD, but are associated with different underlying pathologic processes and carry a significantly worse prognosis.[5] MSA and PSP are the 2 most common APS and account for more than 80% of the APS patients initially misdiagnosed as PD.[4] In addition to parkinsonism, patients with MSA develop autonomic symptoms, such as severe orthostatic hypotension, and cerebellar symptoms, such as ataxia. By contrast, PSP patients develop parkinsonism with early postural instability, falls, and oculomotor abnormalities. Nonetheless, the diagnostic features of APS may not be clinically evident at the early stages of disease. Death is common in MSA and PSP after 7 to 9 years of symptoms, and the pathologic etiologies for both syndromes differ from PD and from one another.[5]

Using FDG PET and spatial covariance analysis, the investigators have recently identified abnormal metabolic patterns for MSA and PSP.[31] By applying strictly defined statistical criteria to the imaging data to define disease-related patterns,[13] the investigators found that these atypical syndromes are each associated with a specific and highly stable metabolic brain network.[32] The MSA-related pattern (MSARP) is characterized by metabolic decreases in the putamen and the cerebellum (**Fig. 2**, *top*). By contrast, the PSP-related pattern (PSPRP) is characterized by metabolic decreases predominately in the upper brainstem and medial prefrontal cortex as well as in the medial thalamus, the caudate nuclei, the anterior cingulate area, and the superior frontal cortex (see **Fig. 2**, *bottom*). In both diseases, pattern expression was found to be stable and significantly elevated ($P<.001$) in patients relative to age-matched healthy control subjects.[32] Pattern expression

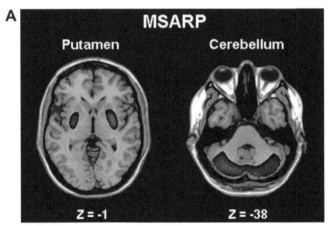

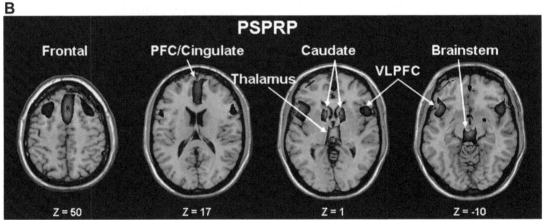

Fig. 2. Spatial covariance patterns associated with atypical parkinsonism. (*A*) Metabolic pattern associated with multiple system atrophy (MSARP) characterized by covarying metabolic decreases in the putamen and cerebellum. (*B*) Metabolic pattern associated with progressive supranuclear palsy (PSPRP) characterized by covarying metabolic decreases in the medial prefrontal cortex (PFC), frontal eye fields, ventrolateral prefrontal cortex (VLPFC), caudate nuclei, medial thalamus, and the upper brainstem. The covariance patterns were overlaid on T1-weighted MR-template images. The displays represent regions that contributed significantly to the network and that were demonstrated to be reliable by bootstrap resampling. Voxels with negative region weights (metabolic decreases) are color-coded blue. (*Reprinted from* Eckert T, Tang C, Ma Y, et al. Abnormal metabolic networks in atypical parkinsonism. Mov Disord 2008;23(5):730,731. Copyright 2008 John Wiley & Sons, Inc, Movement Disorders Society; with permission.)

was also elevated (*P*>.001) in 2 independent patient groups when compared with a prospectively scanned healthy age-matched control group that was different from those originally used to identify the patterns. In MSA patients, the activity of the disease-related pattern in individual subjects increases with disease progression and correlates well with findings at postmortem.[33] Further prospective studies are needed to understand how changes in pattern expression relate to the emergence of symptoms over time. Nonetheless, the preliminary studies suggest the potential utility of the MSARP and the PSPRP as functional imaging biomarkers for these atypical parkinsonian disorders.

DIFFERENTIAL DIAGNOSIS USING PET

Patients with early parkinsonism often present with overlapping signs and symptoms, and only later develop the specific findings needed to make a definitive diagnosis of PD, MSA, or PSP. Accurate clinical diagnosis can often be made only after 2 years of clinical follow-up. Indeed, almost one-quarter of patients initially diagnosed as having PD are ultimately found to have APS on pathology.[4,34] Under ideal circumstances, such patients should be excluded from trials of disease-modifying interventions for PD. Moreover, up to 15% of patients recruited for early, pretreatment clinical trials were found to have a different syndrome on reassessment.[23,35] Diagnostic inclusion criteria for these studies are typically based on clinical evaluation alone, potentially exposing misdiagnosed early APS patients to experimental treatments intended for PD patients. Clinically, patients with APS do not have substantial improvement with dopaminergic medications,[5] and have been found to develop serious complications from standard PD deep brain stimulation (DBS) surgery.[36] For these reasons, accurate diagnosis is critical for patient counseling and treatment decisions. In addition, as new disease-specific treatments emerge targeting the underlying pathophysiology for each of these disorders,[37] there is increased need for early, accurate diagnosis.

Metabolic imaging is a valuable tool to aid in differentiating among these parkinsonian syndromes, particularly in patients with early symptoms. Several FDG PET studies have described characteristic regional patterns of glucose metabolism in PD, MSA, PSP, and corticobasal degeneration (CBD).[38–41] In one study, FDG PET scans from patients with PD, MSA, PSP, and CBD as well as healthy subjects were compared using a voxel-based statistical mapping technique.[39] Maps of regional metabolic differences between patients and controls were used to create characteristic templates for each of these parkinsonian "look-alike" conditions. Disease-defining features of individual scans can be visually matched to the templates, allowing for the best "match" to be made for image classification. A reader with no expertise in PET diagnosis of movement disorders could use this computer-aided visual approach to determine a specific diagnostic category. Indeed, the authors found that using this qualitative technique, the blinded nonexpert's determination agreed with the clinical diagnosis in 92.4% of cases. The accuracy of this template-based approach suggests that it may prove useful clinically, especially when experienced readers of brain FDG PET scans are not readily available.

Highly accurate scan classification can also be achieved using a fully automated pattern quantification approach.[42] In one study, parkinsonian patients with an unclear diagnosis who exhibited normal nigrostriatal dopamine function with ^{18}F-fluorodopa PET were found to have normal PDRP expression, suggesting a diagnosis other than PD.[43] These findings were confirmed when a non-PD diagnosis was established in each patient years later on clinical follow-up. Similarly, prospective PDRP quantification in cerebral perfusion images acquired with ^{99m}Tc ECD SPECT revealed excellent separation of PD and MSA

patients.[44] Furthermore, the application of multiple disease-specific spatial covariance patterns to interrogate individual FDG PET images from early-stage patients can provide an objective and completely user-independent means of classification.[42,45] These findings suggest that disease-related metabolic networks can constitute a powerful adjunct in the differential diagnosis of parkinsonism.

CHANGES IN NETWORK ACTIVITY WITH DISEASE PROGRESSION IN PD

FDG PET has also been found to be useful for monitoring different aspects of disease progression in PD patients. Despite having a unifying underlying pathology, patients with PD can vary significantly with respect to the rate of progression of motor and nonmotor symptoms. For example, motor subtypes of PD, such as tremor-dominant and postural instability with gait difficulty, have been found to have different rates of progression.[46] Moreover, within these subtypes other factors, such as age of onset, can influence the progression of motor impairment.[47] Indeed, these differences can confound clinically based measures of progression rate in the clinical setting and in research trials.

It has recently been shown that FDG PET can provide an objective and accurate means for monitoring disease progression in PD. Longitudinal metabolic imaging studies with PDRP and PDCP quantification have provided unique information concerning functional changes in network activity in patients with early PD.[21] In one study, patients with less than 2 years of clinical symptoms were studied with FDG PET at baseline, 24 months, and 48 months; caudate and putamen dopamine transporter (DAT) binding and clinical motor rating scales (UPDRS) were also measured at each time point. PDRP expression was abnormally elevated in patients at baseline compared with age-matched controls, and continued to increase at each successive time point (**Fig. 3**). These studies also revealed significant correlations between increases in PDRP expression over time and concurrent deterioration in UPDRS motor scores and DAT binding. However, these progression measures were not interchangeable, because less than one-third of the variability in each is explained by the others. Rather, these 3 biomarkers are likely best used in concert, as each captures unique features of disease progression.[12] Larger cross-sectional studies of patients with varying symptom duration corroborate the results of the longitudinal studies. In aggregate, these investigations verify PDRP expression as

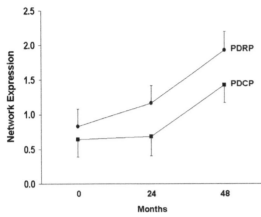

Fig. 3. Longitudinal progression of PD-related pattern expression. Mean network activity at baseline, 24 months, and 48 months. Values for the PD-motor and cognitive spatial covariance patterns (PDRP and PDCP; see **Fig. 1**) were computed at each time point and displayed relative to the mean for 15 age-matched healthy subjects. Network activity increased significantly over time for both patterns ($P<.001$; RMANOVA), with the PDRP progressing faster than the PDCP ($P<.04$). Relative to controls, PDRP activity in the patient group was elevated at all 3 time points, whereas PDCP activity reached abnormal levels only at the final time point. (*Reprinted from* Huang C, Tang C, Feigin A, et al. Changes in network activity with the progression of Parkinson's disease. Brain 2007;130 (Pt 7):1842, Oxford University Press; with permission.)

a sensitive biomarker of PD motor severity throughout the disease course.[13]

Prior to the onset of clinically diagnostic symptoms, there is a suggestion that the PDRP motor network is already abnormal. Neuronal death begins in PD years before symptom onset, and less than 50% of the neurons in the substantia nigra (SN) are functional at the time patients present in the clinic.[48] It is likely that SN neuronal decline is accompanied by compensatory metabolic changes downstream in the CSPTC loops. Because most early patients present with only unilateral appendicular symptoms, the brain hemisphere contralateral to the still asymptomatic side is ideal for studying the "preclinical" condition. Indeed, analysis of "hemispheric" network activity reveals changes in PDRP expression in the asymptomatic hemisphere of early unilateral patients.[49] Longitudinal studies in carriers of susceptibility genes for PD will provide further data concerning changes in metabolic networks prior to the emergence of symptoms.

Longitudinal studies also demonstrate that PDCP expression increases with time in nondemented PD patients, albeit at a different rate of progression from that of the motor pattern.[21]

Whereas the PDRP is elevated in patients at baseline, the PDCP is not elevated until approximately 6 years after symptom onset. Further in the disease course, both the motor and cognitive patterns continue to increase linearly with disease duration, but with different trajectories.[30] The difference in the rate of development of motor and cognitive pattern expression parallels the observed time courses over which motor and cognitive symptoms develop.[2] Increases in PDCP expression are associated not only with symptom duration but also with the degree of cognitive dysfunction that is present in patients. When compared with controls, PD patients exhibit significant increases in PDCP expression prior to the development of cognitive changes on neuropsychological assessment (see **Fig. 3**). As cognitive symptoms emerge, PDCP expression continues to increase in patients exhibiting MCI in single and multiple domains,[29] with further increases as patients develop dementia.[30] These studies demonstrate the specificity of PDCP expression for cognitive dysfunction in PD, and highlight this metabolic network as an objective biomarker for this devastating and progressive disease manifestation.

NETWORK MODULATION WITH PD THERAPY

In the last decade, research efforts have focused on the development of novel surgical and pharmacologic treatment strategies for the motor and nonmotor symptoms of PD. Objective biomarkers that accurately quantify the clinical response to a therapeutic intervention can be extremely useful in determining the efficacy of such new approaches.[6] In this regard, using FDG PET to assess network activity before and during treatment can provide a quantitative index of treatment-mediated changes in brain function at the systems level. Indeed, the quantification of network activity in small therapeutic trials (phases 1 and 2) may be used to objectively screen antiparkinsonian treatments before proceeding with costly and time-consuming efficacy studies.[22,50]

Dopaminergic Therapy

Regional and network changes in metabolic activity have been described in PD patients undergoing treatment with dopaminergic medications.[22,51] Specifically, changes in pallidal metabolism and PDRP expression have been noted with levodopa administration. Indeed, individual differences in the network-level treatment response correlated closely with concurrent changes in UPDRS motor ratings. In the nonmedicated state, regional glucose metabolism is tightly linked to cerebral blood flow.[52] However, a recent study has shown dissociation between cerebral blood flow and glucose metabolism in PD patients during levodopa therapy.[53] This effect was most pronounced in patients with levodopa-induced dyskinesias and was not observed in patients undergoing DBS. The basis of flow-metabolism dissociation with levodopa is thought to reflect vasodilation induced by exogenous dopamine. A better understanding of this mechanism may reveal new targets for treatments aimed at medication-induced dyskinesias.

Whereas many of the motor symptoms of PD improve with dopaminergic therapy, cognitive dysfunction is largely nondopamine responsive. Similarly, PDCP expression is not significantly

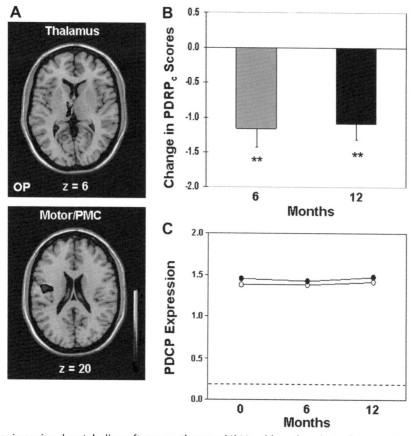

Fig. 4. Changes in regional metabolism after gene therapy. (A) Voxel-based analysis of changes in regional metabolic activity after unilateral STN AAV-GAD gene therapy for advanced PD. After unilateral gene therapy, a significant reduction in metabolism (top) was found in the operated thalamus, involving the ventrolateral and mediodorsal nuclei. The analysis also revealed a significant metabolic increase (bottom) after surgery in the ipsilateral primary motor region (BA 4), which extended into the adjacent lateral premotor cortex (PMC; BA 6). Representative axial T1-weighted MR imaging with merged FDG PET slices; the operated (OP) side is signified on the left. Metabolic increases after surgery are displayed using a red-yellow scale. Metabolic declines are displayed using a blue-purple scale. The displays were thresholded at $P<.05$, corrected for multiple comparisons. (B) Postoperative changes in PDRP activity controlling for the effect of disease progression. These progression-corrected values ($PDRP_c$ scores) reflect the net effect of STN AAV-GAD on network expression for each subject and time point (see text). Relative to baseline, $PDRP_c$ scores declined following gene therapy ($P<.001$, RMANOVA), with significant reductions relative to baseline at both 6 (gray) and 12 (black) months. These changes correlated ($P<.03$) with clinical outcome over the course of the study. $**P<.005$, Bonferroni tests; bars represent standard error. (C) Changes in mean PDCP network activity over time for the operated (filled circles) and the unoperated (open circles) hemispheres. After gene therapy, there was no change in PDCP activity over time in either of the 2 hemispheres ($P = .72$). The dashed line represents one standard error above the normal mean value of zero. (Reprinted from Feigin A, Kaplitt MG, Tang C, et al. Modulation of metabolic brain networks following subthalamic gene therapy for Parkinson's disease. Proc Natl Acad Sci USA 2007;104(49):19560–1, 2007 by The National Academy of Sciences of the USA; with permission.)

changed in patients receiving levodopa.[28] Thus, PDRP expression is an index of the progression of PD motor symptoms and their response to treatment. By contrast, PDCP expression constitutes a marker of the severity of PD cognitive dysfunction in its early stages.

Stereotaxic-Based Surgical Therapy

Modulation of subthalamic nucleus (STN) activity with DBS has been used to produce clinical improvement in PD patients comparable to that achieved with dopaminergic drugs. Indeed, STN ablation and STN DBS are thought to ameliorate PD motor symptoms by mechanisms similar to those of dopamine therapy.[54] Intraoperative microelectrode recordings during STN DBS electrode placement in PD patients have revealed an increase in the mean firing rate of STN neurons,[55] which is correlated significantly with PDRP expression.[56] This increase suggests that network activity might be modulated by surgical interventions in this region. Indeed, STN DBS is associated with significant reductions in PDRP expression, correlating with clinical changes in motor function.[22]

Although both dopamine therapy and STN DBS similarly suppress PDRP expression, the effects on network activity are not additive.[22] Data from patients with both therapies suggest that it is unlikely for combination therapy to lower network activity beyond a naturally defined "floor." Similarly, a recent study using FDG PET addressed changes in PDRP expression after STN "microlesion,"[57] defined as the change in network activity that occurs after STN microelectrode recording and electrode insertion but before STN stimulation. Regional changes in glucose metabolism were evident in regions receiving either direct or indirect input from the STN, such as the putamen, globus pallidus, and the ventral thalamus.[56] However, the magnitude of these changes was smaller compared with changes seen with therapeutic STN lesioning (subthalamotomy)[58] or DBS.[22] These findings imply that upper and lower thresholds exist for therapeutic PDRP modulation, defining the minimum and maximum functional changes achievable at the STN target site.

Gene Transfer Therapy

Gene transfer therapy is a novel form of treatment for neurodegenerative disease such as PD.[50] Small, well-designed phase 1 trials are critical for evaluating the safety and tolerability of this technique. Moreover, neuroimaging techniques such as FDG PET can be invaluable as objective in vivo biomarkers for the assessment of treatment response. In a recent phase I clinical trial, the authors used this approach to measure the safety, tolerability, and potential efficacy of an adeno-associated virus (AAV)-borne glutamic acid decarboxylase (GAD) gene transferred into the STN of PD patients.[8,9,50] FDG PET was performed on patients at baseline, 6 months after, and 12 months after unilateral gene transfer therapy for the STN. There were significant reductions in thalamic metabolism on the operated side as well as concurrent metabolic increases in ipsilateral motor and premotor cortical regions (**Fig. 4**A). PDRP activity on the operated side was significantly reduced at 6 months with continued reduction at 12 months (see **Fig. 4**B). This change correlated with improvement in clinical motor UPDRS ratings contralateral to the operated side.[8] By contrast, there was no change in PDCP activity or neuropsychological rates at any time point (see **Fig. 4**C). These studies indicate the use of FDG PET and network analysis as an objective, blinded biomarker for use in open-label phase 1 clinical trials for the development of novel therapies in PD.

SUMMARY

Spatial covariance analysis of metabolic imaging data from patients with neurodegenerative disorders has provided valuable insights into the pathophysiology of these diseases. This approach has been used recently with FDG PET to characterize and measure disease-related metabolic patterns as specific network biomarkers for differential diagnosis and the assessment of responses to therapy. For instance, distinct metabolic patterns associated with the motor and cognitive manifestations of PD have been used to assess network modulation after gene therapy. FDG PET investigations are being conducted to assess the accuracy of early differential diagnosis of parkinsonism based solely on pattern analysis. Other studies are being planned to validate disease-related patterns for APS such as MSA and PSP. Validated metabolic networks for these atypical syndromes will aid in the development of novel therapeutic targets for these refractory conditions. Overall, metabolic imaging with FDG PET in conjunction with pattern analysis is likely to enhance diagnostic accuracy and facilitate the development of new treatments for PD and related disorders.

ACKNOWLEDGMENTS

The authors wish to thank Toni Flanagan for her valuable editorial assistance.

REFERENCES

1. de Rijk MC, Breteler MM, Graveland GA, et al. Prevalence of Parkinson's disease in the elderly: the Rotterdam Study. Neurology 1995;45(12):2143–6.
2. Hely MA, Morris JG, Reid WG, et al. Sydney multicenter study of Parkinson's disease: non-L-dopa-responsive problems dominate at 15 years. Mov Disord 2005;20(2):190–9.
3. Hely MA, Reid WG, Adena MA, et al. The Sydney multicenter study of Parkinson's disease: the inevitability of dementia at 20 years. Mov Disord 2008; 23(6):837–44.
4. Hughes AJ, Daniel SE, Ben-Shlomo Y, et al. The accuracy of diagnosis of parkinsonian syndromes in a specialist movement disorder service. Brain 2002;125(Pt 4):861–70.
5. O'Sullivan SS, Massey LA, Williams DR, et al. Clinical outcomes of progressive supranuclear palsy and multiple system atrophy. Brain 2008;131(Pt 5): 1362–72.
6. Poston KL, Eidelberg D. Network biomarkers for the diagnosis and treatment of movement disorders. Neurobiol Dis 2009;35(2):141–7.
7. Freed CR, Greene PE, Breeze RE, et al. Transplantation of embryonic dopamine neurons for severe Parkinson's disease. N Engl J Med 2001;344(10):710–9.
8. Feigin A, Kaplitt MG, Tang C, et al. Modulation of metabolic brain networks after subthalamic gene therapy for Parkinson's disease. Proc Natl Acad Sci U S A 2007;104(49):19559–64.
9. Kaplitt MG, Feigin A, Tang C, et al. Safety and tolerability of gene therapy with an adeno-associated virus (AAV) borne GAD gene for Parkinson's disease: an open label, phase I trial. Lancet 2007; 369(9579):2097–105.
10. Eidelberg D, Takikawa S, Moeller JR, et al. Striatal hypometabolism distinguishes striatonigral degeneration from Parkinson's disease. Ann Neurol 1993; 33(5):518–27.
11. Alexander GE, Moeller JR. Application of the scaled subprofile model to functional imaging in neuropsychiatric disorders: a principal component approach to modeling brain function in disease. Hum Brain Mapp 1994;2:1–16.
12. Eckert T, Tang C, Eidelberg D. Assessment of the progression of Parkinson's disease: a metabolic network approach. Lancet Neurol 2007;6(10):926–32.
13. Eidelberg D. Metabolic brain networks in neurodegenerative disorders: a functional imaging approach. Trends Neurosci 2009;32(10):548–57.
14. Habeck C, Foster NL, Perneczky R, et al. Multivariate and univariate neuroimaging biomarkers of Alzheimer's disease. Neuroimage 2008;40(4):1503–15.
15. Feigin A, Tang C, Ma Y, et al. Thalamic metabolism and symptom onset in preclinical Huntington's disease. Brain 2007;130(Pt 11):2858–67.
16. DeLong MR, Wichmann T. Circuits and circuit disorders of the basal ganglia. Arch Neurol 2007;64(1): 20–4.
17. Ma Y, Tang C, Moeller JR, et al. Abnormal regional brain function in Parkinson's disease: truth or fiction? Neuroimage 2009;45(2):260–6.
18. Eidelberg D, Moeller JR, Dhawan V, et al. The metabolic topography of parkinsonism. J Cereb Blood Flow Metab 1994;14(5):783–801.
19. Eidelberg D, Moeller JR, Kazumata K, et al. Metabolic correlates of pallidal neuronal activity in Parkinson's disease. Brain 1997;120(Pt 8):1315–24.
20. Ma Y, Tang C, Spetsieris PG, et al. Abnormal metabolic network activity in Parkinson's disease: test-retest reproducibility. J Cereb Blood Flow Metab 2007; 27(3):597–605.
21. Huang C, Tang C, Feigin A, et al. Changes in network activity with the progression of Parkinson's disease. Brain 2007;130(Pt 7):1834–46.
22. Asanuma K, Tang C, Ma Y, et al. Network modulation in the treatment of Parkinson's disease. Brain 2006; 129(Pt 10):2667–78.
23. Fahn S, Oakes D, Shoulson I, et al. Levodopa and the progression of Parkinson's disease. N Engl J Med 2004;351(24):2498–508.
24. Antonini A, Moeller JR, Nakamura T, et al. The metabolic anatomy of tremor in Parkinson's disease. Neurology 1998;51(3):803–10.
25. Isaias IU, Marotta G, Hirano S, et al. Imaging essential tremor. Mov Disord, in press.
26. Levy G, Tang MX, Louis ED, et al. The association of incident dementia with mortality in PD. Neurology 2002;59(11):1708–13.
27. Bosboom JL, Stoffers D, Wolters E. Cognitive dysfunction and dementia in Parkinson's disease. J Neural Transm 2004;111(10–11):1303–15.
28. Huang C, Mattis P, Tang C, et al. Metabolic brain networks associated with cognitive function in Parkinson's disease. Neuroimage 2007;34(2):714–23.
29. Huang C, Mattis P, Perrine K, et al. Metabolic abnormalities associated with mild cognitive impairment in Parkinson disease. Neurology 2008;70(16 Pt 2): 1470–7.
30. Poston KL, Mattis P, Tang C, et al. Metabolic abnormalities associated with progressive cognitive dysfunction in Parkinson's disease. Neurology 2009;72(11):A114.
31. Eckert T, Edwards C. The application of network mapping in differential diagnosis of parkinsonian disorders. Clin Neurosci Res 2007;6:359–66.
32. Eckert T, Tang C, Ma Y, et al. Abnormal metabolic networks in atypical parkinsonism. Mov Disord 2008;23(5):727–33.
33. Poston KL, Tang C, Eckert T, et al. Longitudinal changes in regional metabolism and network activity in multiple system atrophy. Neurology 2009; 72(Suppl 3):A67.

34. Hughes AJ, Daniel SE, Kilford L, et al. Accuracy of clinical diagnosis of idiopathic Parkinson's disease: a clinico-pathological study of 100 cases. J Neurol Neurosurg Psychiatr 1992;55(3):181–4.

35. Jankovic J, Rajput AH, McDermott MP, et al. The evolution of diagnosis in early Parkinson disease. Parkinson study group. Arch Neurol 2000;57(3): 369–72.

36. Shih LC, Tarsy D. Deep brain stimulation for the treatment of atypical parkinsonism. Mov Disord 2007;22(15):2149–55.

37. Zhou J, Yu Q, Zou T. Alternative splicing of exon 10 in the tau gene as a target for treatment of tauopathies. BMC Neurosci 2008;9(Suppl 2):S10.

38. Feng T, Wang Y, Ouyang Q, et al. Comparison of cerebral glucose metabolism between multiple system atrophy Parkinsonian type and Parkinson's disease. Neurol Res 2008;30(4):377–82.

39. Eckert T, Barnes A, Dhawan V, et al. FDG PET in the differential diagnosis of parkinsonian disorders. Neuroimage 2005;26(3):912–21.

40. Juh R, Pae CU, Lee CU, et al. Voxel based comparison of glucose metabolism in the differential diagnosis of the multiple system atrophy using statistical parametric mapping. Neurosci Res 2005; 52(3):211–9.

41. Otsuka M, Kuwabara Y, Ichiya Y, et al. Differentiating between multiple system atrophy and Parkinson's disease by positron emission tomography with ^{18}F-dopa and ^{18}F-FDG. Ann Nucl Med 1997; 11(3):251–7.

42. Spetsieris PG, Ma Y, Dhawan V, et al. Differential diagnosis of parkinsonian syndromes using PCA-based functional imaging features. Neuroimage 2009;45(4):1241–52.

43. Eckert T, Feigin A, Lewis DE, et al. Regional metabolic changes in parkinsonian patients with normal dopaminergic imaging. Mov Disord 2007;22(2): 167–73.

44. Eckert T, Van Laere K, Tang C, et al. Quantification of Parkinson's disease-related network expression with ECD SPECT. Eur J Nucl Med Mol Imaging 2007; 34(4):496–501.

45. Tang CC, Poston KL, Eckert T, et al. Differential diagnosis of parkinsonism: a metabolic imaging study using pattern analysis. Lancet Neurol 2010;9(2): 149–58.

46. Alves G, Larsen JP, Emre M, et al. Changes in motor subtype and risk for incident dementia in Parkinson's disease. Mov Disord 2006;21(8):1123–30.

47. Alves G, Wentzel-Larsen T, Aarsland D, et al. Progression of motor impairment and disability in Parkinson disease: a population-based study. Neurology 2005;65(9):1436–41.

48. Bernheimer H, Birkmayer W, Hornykiewicz O, et al. Brain dopamine and the syndromes of Parkinson and Huntington. Clinical, morphological and neurochemical correlations. J Neurol Sci 1973;20: 415–55.

49. Tang CC, Poston KL, Dhawan V, et al. Abnormalities in metabolic network activity precede the onset of motor symptoms in Parkinson's disease. J Neurosci 2010;30(3):1049–56.

50. Feigin A, Eidelberg D. Gene transfer therapy for neurodegenerative disorders. Mov Disord 2007; 22(9):1223–8.

51. Feigin A, Fukuda M, Dhawan V, et al. Metabolic correlates of levodopa response in Parkinson's disease. Neurology 2001;57(11):2083–8.

52. Raichle ME. Behind the scenes of functional brain imaging: a historical and physiological perspective. Proc Natl Acad Sci U S A 1998;95(3):765–72.

53. Hirano S, Asanuma K, Ma Y, et al. Dissociation of metabolic and neurovascular responses to levodopa in the treatment of Parkinson's disease. J Neurosci 2008;28(16):4201–9.

54. Vingerhoets FJ, Villemure JG, Temperli P, et al. Subthalamic DBS replaces levodopa in Parkinson's disease: two-year follow-up. Neurology 2002;58(3): 396–401.

55. Steigerwald F, Potter M, Herzog J, et al. Neuronal activity of the human subthalamic nucleus in the parkinsonian and nonparkinsonian state. J Neurophysiol 2008;100(5):2515–24.

56. Lin TP, Carbon M, Tang C, et al. Metabolic correlates of subthalamic nucleus activity in Parkinson's disease. Brain 2008;131(5):1373–80.

57. Pourfar M, Tang C, Lin T, et al. Assessing the microlesion effect of subthalamic deep brain stimulation surgery with FDG PET. J Neurosurg 2009;110(6): 1278–82.

58. Trost M, Su S, Su P, et al. Network modulation by the subthalamic nucleus in the treatment of Parkinson's disease. Neuroimage 2006;31(1):301–7.

SPECT and PET in Atypical Parkinsonism

John P. Seibyl, MD

KEYWORDS

• Parkinson disease • Biomarkers
• Dopaminergic imaging • Movement disorders

THE SPECTRUM OF MOVEMENT DISORDERS

Parkinson disease (PD) is the prototypic movement disorder originally described by James Parkinson, and it accounts for about 80% of a group of related degenerative motor disorders collectively referred to as the parkinsonisms, Parkinson spectrum disorders, or Parkinson plus disorders, terms which are used interchangeably throughout this article. In addition to idiopathic PD, these disorders include progressive supranuclear palsy (PSP), multiple system atrophy (MSA), and corticobasal degeneration (CBD). All of the neurodegenerative disorders under this rubric are characterized by both motor and nonmotor symptoms, which progress over time, but are distinguished by different pathophysiologic underpinnings, clinical prognosis, rate of symptom progression, associated clinical phenomenology, and treatment.[1,2] Secondary parkinsonism refers to Parkinson-like motor impairment occurring in the context of toxic, infectious, metabolic, vascular, neoplastic, drug-induced, or other insults to motor circuits resulting in tremor, bradykinesia, or other Parkinson-like manifestations. In addition, other neurodegenerative disorders may be confused with the parkinsonisms, including dementia with Lewy bodies (DLB), Alzheimer disease, Huntington disease, or familial neurodegenerative disease (Table 1).

This wide array of disorders with overlapping clinical phenomenology can provide a significant diagnostic challenge, particularly early in the course of illness when symptoms may be subtle or only partially manifested. For example, the initial motor symptoms of idiopathic PD occur generally on one side of the body and gradually progress to the salient features of bradykinesia, tremor, and disturbance of gait involving both sides of the body. These cardinal features of PD develop later than nonmotor symptoms. Nonmotor manifestations are less well understood and include loss of olfaction, altered bowel function, and sleep disturbances.[1,3–6] Later nonmotor manifestations include cognitive impairment, affective restriction, and frank depression. These later symptoms are complicated by medication treatments with agents such as levodopa, which in addition to almost invariably producing dopaminergic complications, such as dyskinesias and abrupt on-off motor fluctuations, can also cause delusional ideation and paranoia, hallucinations, and obsessionality.[7] Hence, for even the relatively more common idiopathic PD, the changing panoply of symptoms over time provides a potential source of confusion for the community neurologist or primary care physician, with many viable alternative diagnoses.[2,8] It is not surprising that studies indicate the accuracy of clinical diagnosis to be low in new-onset patients, whether diagnosed by general practitioners, community neurologists, or movement disorder specialists. Such studies demonstrate that primary care physicians incorrectly diagnose parkinsonism in about one-third of patients, whereas movement disorder specialists misdiagnose PD about 10% to 12% of the time. Similarly, in large phase 3 clinical studies, more than 10% of de novo PD patients who meet operational diagnostic criteria as assessed by a movement disorder neurologist are misdiagnosed.[9] Hence, diagnosis remains a clear challenge.

Distinguishing between the Parkinson plus disorders, essential tremor, secondary parkinsonisms, DLB, and even look-alike Alzheimer disease is important not only from the perspective of treatment

Institute for Neurodegenerative Disorders, Molecular Neuroimaging, LLC, Yale University School of Medicine, 60 Temple Street, 8B, New Haven, CT 06510, USA
E-mail address: jseibyl@indd.org

PET Clin 5 (2010) 65–74
doi:10.1016/j.cpet.2010.02.005

Table 1
Differential diagnosis of movement disorders

Parkinson spectrum disorders	Idiopathic PD
	PSP
	MSA
	Familial PD
Secondary parkinsonism	Vascular
	Infectious
	Neoplastic
	Traumatic
	Drug-induced

DLB
Essential tremor
Psychogenic PD
Huntington disease
Frontotemporal dementia
Alzheimer dementia

but also for appropriate prognosis and planning. The movement disorder specialists and well-versed clinicians rely on several clinical features to distinguish between the parkinsonisms and other neurodegenerative disorders, including age of onset, presence of gaze palsies, acuity of onset, onset of postural instability and dysautonomias, hallucinations, the presence and type of tremor, timing of dementia onset, ataxia, apraxia, symmetry of onset, and response to dopamine replacement treatment. The most reliable aid to clinical diagnosis is the ability to track a patient's symptoms and response to medication over several months. Nonetheless, even in this scenario, studies consistently show about 11% to 14% misdiagnosis rate by movement disorder specialists in evaluating new-onset patients with suspected PD.[9]

In this context, molecular imaging may assist clinical assessment and ultimately management. The roles of molecular imaging are only partially established and remain reliant on ongoing research to integrate appropriate clinical imaging protocols and tracers into management algorithms.[10–12] Nonetheless, imaging techniques are currently being used to aid in the differential diagnosis of PD, identification of patients at risk for movement disorders, screening of patients into large clinical trials, and in monitoring the efficacy of novel treatments. In particular, there is extensive interest in the next generation of therapeutics for the patients with Parkinson syndrome whose intent is to modify the ongoing course of illness in addition to ameliorating debilitating motor and nonmotor symptoms.[13]

Both the elaboration of new treatments and the intelligent use of imaging tools require a sophisticated knowledge of the pathologic changes in brain associated with each disorder. Although seemingly straightforward, in fact, this very active area of research demonstrates significant overlap in the type of pathophysiologic change occurring in these disorders. Nonetheless, even as the pathologic patterns in brain are being elaborated in PD and related disorders, there remain opportunities for neuroimaging measures to exploit the specificity of radiopharmaceuticals to support clinical and research applications. Hence, the potential roles of the nuclear imaging modalities depend on the current understanding of the pathologic changes occurring in these disorders and the research community's ability to develop and validate radiopharmaceutical agents for specific brain targets.

DOPAMINERGIC IMAGING IN THE DIAGNOSIS OF PARKINSONISM AND RELATED DISORDERS

Much work with positron emission tomography (PET) and single-photon emission computed tomography (SPECT) in the movement disorders has focused on the dopamine system. The discovery of marked degeneration of dopaminergic neurons within the substantia nigra, which project to the striatum (caudate and putamen), was made nearly a century ago. This finding has provided both a rationale for symptomatic therapy as well as a target for imaging agents. There have been at least 3 different presynaptic dopaminergic targets that are used successfully to interrogate the dopamine system, with several radioligands for each: the dopamine transporter (^{123}I-FP-CIT [DaTSCAN] and many others),[14] the vesicular transporter (^{11}C-VMAT2, ^{18}F-AV-133),[15] and dopamine metabolism (^{18}F-dopa) (**Fig. 1**).[16,17] Although each of these targets represents a different aspect of presynaptic dopamine function, there exists now several decades' worth of research and clinical application in assessing dopamine system changes with these targets to differentially diagnose, monitor, and screen patients with movement disorders. The clinical data do not as yet indicate whether one modality or target is superior in aiding the diagnosis or monitoring the disease.[18] Furthermore, it is not clear how well SPECT and PET quantitative measures reflect actual neuronal cell loss. Nonetheless, each of these techniques have consistently shown in idiopathic PD a left-right asymmetric signal loss that corresponds with motor asymmetry, greater reductions in the putamen relative to the caudate, correlation with quantitative outcome measures and disease staging in cross-sectional studies, and finally, progressive imaging signal loss that is consistent with ongoing neurodegeneration in longitudinal studies.[19–21]

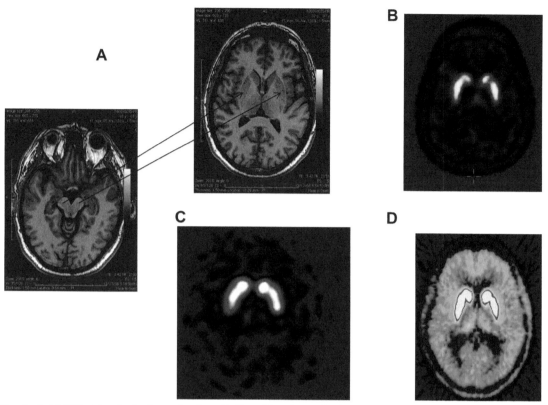

Fig. 1. Axial MRI at level of substantia nigra (*left*) and basal ganglia (*right*) demonstrating projections of nigral dopamine neurons (Panel A). Panels B, C, and D demonstrate 3 different presynaptic dopaminergic targets in healthy human subjects. Panel B shows striata imaged with the VMAT2 agent, ^{18}F AV133, panel C shows dopamine transporter imaging with [123]I β-CIT, and panel D indicates dopa metabolism with ^{18}F-FDOPA. A similar pattern of uptake is demonstrated despite different presynaptic targets and scintigraphic modality.

Although the great bulk of imaging studies with presynaptic dopaminergic approaches have been in idiopathic PD, there have been several studies evaluating the clinical utility and pathophysiologic changes of these imaging measures in patients with Parkinson syndrome. From the perspective of differential diagnosis, all Parkinson syndromes involve dopamine neuronal degeneration, and hence, presynaptic dopaminergic imaging does not easily discriminate idiopathic PD from the Parkinson plus disorders, such as PSP, MSA, and CBD. All patients with these disorders demonstrate markedly reduced striatal uptake, with a tendency to exhibit less left-right and anteroposterior striatal asymmetry compared with idiopathic PD.[22] However, there is a significant overlap between the scintigraphic findings of all these disorders, making presynaptic dopaminergic imaging alone inadequate for discriminating between the Parkinson spectrum disorders. Hence, routine presynaptic dopaminergic functional imaging for differential diagnosis of these disorders is not indicated (**Fig. 2**).

In this case, studies evaluating other aspects of dopaminergic function including postsynaptic receptor binding and measures of intrasynaptic dopamine function have been evaluated as an aid to differential diagnosis. In particular, PSP and MSA do demonstrate reductions in postsynaptic D_2/D_3 dopamine-receptor densities. In idiopathic PD, postsynaptic receptor density is either normal or mildly elevated in early disease.[22] However, the clinical incorporation of routine protocols for assessing pre- and postsynaptic dopamine-receptor function in the differential diagnosis of Parkinson syndromes has not been commonly applied, because again there is overlap among the imaging findings of PD spectrum patients and the availability of the radiotracers for routine clinical use is severely limited in many regions of the world.

Another approach is to assess the dynamics of dopamine release into the synapse. This has been studied in idiopathic PD by the use of reversible-bound PET tracers, such as ^{11}C raclopride, or SPECT tracers, such as ^{123}I IBZM. It is possible to

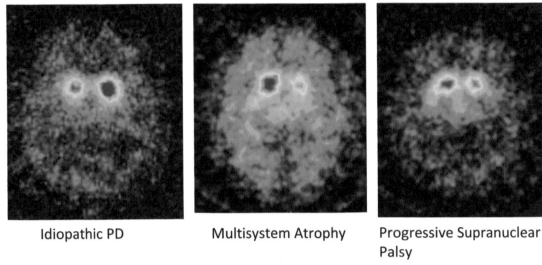

Idiopathic PD   Multisystem Atrophy   Progressive Supranuclear Palsy

Fig. 2. Patients with Idiopathic PD, MSA, and PSP imaged with [123]I β-CIT, a marker of the dopamine transporter, showed similar reductions in striatal uptake across these disorders, with more involvement in putamen compared with caudate and left-right asymmetry. (*Adapted from* van Heertum R, Tikofsky R, Ichise M. Functional cerebral SPECT and PET imaging, Philadelphis: Wolters Kluwer, 2010; with permission.)

image synaptic dopamine release by assessing the degree of striatal signal loss occurring after challenging the patient with drugs that produce transient increases in dopamine release into the synapse, including D-amphetamine or L-dopa. These agents do not act directly on the postsynaptic D_2/D_3 receptor but rather increase the endogenous dopamine level, which then competes with the radiotracer for binding to the receptor, causing reduction in specifically bound radiotracers. For example, after intravenous administration of L-dopa (3 mg/kg) into patients with PD, there is a 6% to 18% displacement in ^{11}C raclopride binding. Another study used this technique with ^{11}C raclopride PET and an oral L-dopa (250 mg) challenge to show that patients with significant on-off symptom fluctuations demonstrated a 7% reduction of striatal binding at 1 hour but returned to baseline levels after 4 hours, whereas those patients without medication-induced motor fluctuations had a persisting effect of L-dopa even after 4 hours.[23–26] Hence, the dynamic response to dopamine replacement therapy is different among patients with idiopathic PD. Similar studies have been performed using constant infusion methods with the SPECT tracer ^{123}I IBZM. As yet, this approach has not been extensively applied to assess dopamine dynamics in other parkinsonisms, and it should be done with the caveat that underlying alterations in postsynaptic D_2/D_3 receptors' sites make the interpretation of findings more complicated.

From the perspective of the most practical clinical utility, dopamine system imaging returns us to presynaptic dopaminergic imaging in which PET or SPECT biomarkers continue to be used in the differential diagnosis between Parkinson syndromes and other disease entities such as essential tremor, drug-induced parkinsonism, vascular parkinsonism, psychogenic parkinsonism, or dementia spectrum disorders, which may mimic some features of the parkinsonisms, particularly early in the course of illness. In addition, the use of presynaptic dopaminergic imaging with SPECT dopamine-transporter ligands, such as ^{123}I-FP-CIT, has been particularly successful in distinguishing between Lewy body dementia (DLB) and Alzheimer dementia, in which the former has significant reductions in striatal dopamine transporters, which remain unaffected in patients with Alzheimer disease (**Table 2**).

One critique of current approaches to differential diagnosis lies in questions as to the actual clinical need for this information. The argument goes that there is little intrinsic value from a management standpoint to understand whether a patient has idiopathic PD or one of the related PD spectrum disorders. Evaluation and treatment may initially be the same, although response to dopaminergic therapies is either poor or has diminishing benefit, as in the case of PSP and MSA. Countering this is the argument that the different clinical course and responses to the treatment of Parkinson spectrum disorders requires accurate nosologic

Table 2				
Imaging findings in Parkinson, Parkinson spectrum, and other neurodegenerative disorders				
	Presynaptic Dopamine	Post synaptic Dopamine	Amyloid	Cardiac MIBG
Idiopathic PD	Decreased	Up or NL	NL	Decreased
PSP	Decreased	Decreased		NL
MSA	Decreased	Decreased		NL
Essential tremor	NL	NL	NL	NL
DLB	Decreased		Increased	Decreased
Alzheimer disease	NL	NL	Increased	NL
Drug-induced PD	NL	NL	NL	NL

Abbreviations: MIBG, metaiodobenzylguanidine; NL, normal.

classification, because this is extremely useful to the patient, physician, and the family for planning based on a reasonable understanding of what to expect over time as the disease inexorably progresses.

Another way of looking at this is not from the perspective of differential clinical diagnosis but from the perspective of pathologic diagnosis. PET and SPECT imaging provide only the information about the status of a brain target. P It may be that pathophysiologic information provided by presynaptic dopaminergic imaging, although of limited value in the differential diagnosis of Parkinson spectrum disorders, is important in the early determination of alterations occurring in the brain reflecting a neurodegenerative process of dopamine systems, regardless of etiology. It is accepted that therapeutic interventions designed to modify the course of disease and slow down the progression of illness are best initiated at the very early stages, during which there is most potential for neuronal salvage. It may not matter whether the patient is diagnosed with idiopathic PD or other Parkinson spectrum disorders. The mechanisms that underlie the disease progression may be similar. In which case, the demonstration of a dopaminergic deficit without regard to the precise diagnosis remains relevant.

Much recent research in the use of presynaptic dopaminergic imaging biomarkers has been in the area of early diagnosis. Specifically, how is it possible to use imaging to identify patients at the very early stages of the disease even before the expression of the clinical criteria required to make the diagnosis become manifest? And what window does imaging provide in identifying pathophysiologic change occurring potentially years before diagnosis that might be relevant for therapeutic intervention?

It is known that when patients with idiopathic PD first present to their community neurologist or movement disorder specialist, imaging measures consistently show 35% to 50% signal loss in the most affected putamen.[27] In addition, as these patients present with asymmetric symptoms, in which one side of their body is clinically normal while the other demonstrates tremor, bradykinesia, and other symptoms, presynaptic dopamine system imaging reveals bilateral changes, with greater involvement in the contralateral side to symptom expression. Hence, presynaptic dopaminergic markers are exquisitely sensitive to changes occurring upstream from peripheral motor pathways and their presence is an early identifiable finding. But it is not understood how early these striatal deficits can be best detected and what clinical role does the ability to see these changes with PET or SPECT biomarkers play in the clinical management of patients who either have a tentative diagnosis or are at risk for the diagnosis based on still inchoate clinical symptoms, genetic predisposition, or other factors.

What may be ultimately possible is the transition from a model of symptomatic treatment of clinically characterized disorders to a diagnosis based on molecular biomarkers (imaging or otherwise) and treatments designed to influence those pathologic biochemical processes without regard to specific clinical diagnosis or even characteristic symptoms. Specifically, the model is molecular imaging for molecular diagnosis to guide molecular treatment. This may result in a very different understanding of the disease but ultimately could have the greatest impact on the course of a neurodegenerative illness.

However, such an approach is speculative and currently unsupported by longitudinal studies of imaging in large cohorts of at-risk patients. In addition, until a proven disease-modifying agent in PD and related disorders becomes available, there is less value to tracking down and characterizing patients at risk. The challenge is to have clinically valid approaches in place for the selection of those patients who might benefit from disease-modifying interventions when such are available. This places the onus on nuclear physicians to make early and accurate molecular diagnoses using imaging biomarkers.

NONDOPAMINERGIC IMAGING IN THE DIFFERENTIAL DIAGNOSIS OF MOVEMENT DISORDERS

Although the dopamine system is a target for clinical and research molecular imaging in idiopathic PD and related disorders, these disorders are clearly more complex and subtle, involving a wider range of aberrations in monoaminergic and nonaminergic neuronal systems, abnormal protein deposition, and neuroinflammation, suggesting potentially useful imaging tools for interrogation of these aspects of altered brain function. Even nigrostriatal dysfunction, which is only one aspect of a complicated pattern of brain pathology in the parkinsonisms, has an effect across multiple brain neurochemical system and circuits, which react to, compensate for, and in some instances, exacerbate this deficit. To this end, the use of FDG-PET imaging as a means of assessing the metabolic consequences of neurodegeneration has been shown to assist in the differential diagnosis of the parkinsonisms.[28] Analyses of FDG-PET results demonstrate specific abnormal spatial covariance patterns in idiopathic PD (PD-related motor pattern [PDRP]), PD patients with cognitive dysfunction (PD-related cognitive pattern), and other Parkinson spectrum disorders related to functional alterations in different clusters of neuronal circuits.[29] Furthermore, because cerebral metabolism and blood flow are normally coupled, these covariance measurements can also be made on cerebral perfusion studies with either PET (^{15}O water) or SPECT (99m TC-ECD). PDRP is stable and reproducible within individual patients,[30] correlates with clinical ratings, increases with progressing disease, and is sensitive to medication treatment.[31,32] Recent studies have shown that metabolic network approaches are useful in differentiating PD from other parkinsonisms.[33] Current studies are assessing these techniques with an eye to the practical application in the assessment of patients with suspected movement disorders. The value of such an approach lies in the potential for an objective method using readily available ^{18}F FDG-PET, which can identify not only patterns in the parkinsonisms but also clusters of symptoms, including early cognitive changes and metabolic patterns across disease entities.

Another target of interest in the differential diagnosis of PD lies not in the brain but in the heart. Several studies have been conducted evaluating the cardiac accumulation of ^{123}I metaiodobenzylguanidine (MIBG), a marker of myocardial sympathetic nervous system integrity. This agent is used clinically for the detection of neuroendocrine tumors. It is possible to derive a simple semiquantitative outcome measure, the heart to mediastinal ratio (H/M), determined on early and delayed planar gamma camera acquisitions, which distinguishes PD from MSA and PSP. H/M ratios are low in PD and other Lewy body neurodegenerative disease (ie, DLB), whereas the ratios are within the normal range in the parkinsonisms.[34–38] As discussed earlier, it is very difficult to use presynaptic dopamine imaging methods alone to discriminate idiopathic PD from parkinsonisms, but it may be feasible to use a combination of imaging approaches to establish this differential diagnosis (**Fig. 3**).

Another more experimental imaging biomarker, which holds some theoretical promise in evaluating PD is an agent that assesses neuroinflammatory processes. Inflammation is thought to be generically involved in neurodegenerative disorders. Pathologic examination of the brains of patients with PD demonstrates the presence of activated microglia in both subcortical and cortical regions. These microglia represent an inflammatory response to the disease and may be quite relevant to ongoing cell loss and progression of symptoms. When microglia are recruited into an area of inflammation, potential cytotoxic substances including cytokines and reactive oxygen compounds (hydrogen peroxide and superoxide) are produced. Cytokines themselves activate microglia, potentially setting up a positive feedback mechanism.

Activated microglia elaborate a receptor, the translocator protein (TSPO, 18 kDa) found on outer mitochondrial membranes, also known as the peripheral benzodiazepine receptor. Radiolabeled compounds targeting this receptor provide a measure of the location and degree of inflammation.[39–41]

By far, most experience in human studies has been with ^{11}C PK11195, which has been evaluated in studies of Alzheimer disease, PD, and related disorders. PET imaging using ^{11}C PK11195 shows focally increased uptake in Alzheimer disease, PD, MSA, cortical-basal ganglionic degeneration, and PSP. In PD there is increased ^{11}C PK11195 uptake in the pons, basal ganglia, and frontal and temporal cortical regions. Longitudinal assessments of PD in limited numbers of subjects suggest that neuroinflammatory changes remain stable. Furthermore, in idiopathic PD, changes

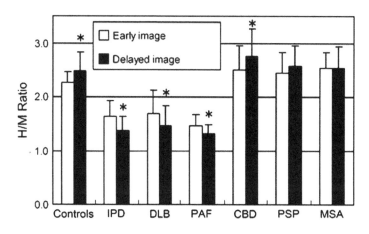

Fig. 3. Mean H/M ratios obtained on early and delayed planar imaging with ^{123}I MIBG in controls (n = 16), idiopathic PD(IPD, n = 130), DLB (n = 21), pure autonomic failure (PAF, n = 6), CBD (n = 9), PSP (n = 11), and MSA (n = 11) demonstrate reduction in IPD, DLB, and PAF, but not in other Parkinson spectrum disorders. Asterisks indicate significant differences within each patient cohort between early and late ratios, with IPD, DLB, and PAF groups showing reduced late ratios and faster washout compared with other groups. (*From* Kashihara K, Ohno M, Kawada S, et al. Reduced cardiac uptake and enhanced washout of 123I-MIBG in pure autonomic failure occurs conjointly with Parkinson's disease and dementia with Lewy bodies. J Nucl Med 2006;47(7):1099–101; with permission.)

are widespread but do not correlate with clinical severity or presynaptic dopaminergic imaging with ^{18}F-FDOPA PET.[42] Patients with PSP demonstrate significantly increased ^{11}C PK11195 uptake not only in the basal ganglia but also in the midbrain, frontal lobe, and cerebellum.[43] It is too early to know whether there will be robust specificity in the regional pattern of brain uptake relevant to differential diagnosis and, if so, whether there will be a clinical role for imaging this brain target. It has been suggested that neuroinflammation in itself is a target for treatment of neurodegenerative disorders, and hence, a good biomarker of this process could be of some clinical utility. The search for better radiopharmaceuticals for interrogation of TSPO has led to the recent development of both ^{18}F and ^{123}I radiotracers. These are currently in initial human validation studies.

Other nonscintigraphic neuroimaging approaches, such as voxel-based morphometry or diffusion tensor imaging, are also in the early stages of research for evaluating patients with PD and parkinsonism,[44–48] and they may provide additional information relevant to the diagnosis based on morphometric measures or functional disruption in the integrity of networks and nerve tracts. As yet, there are limited data on the utility of these approaches in early detection, at-risk assessment, differential diagnosis, or disease monitoring.

IDENTIFYING NEW TARGETS AND IMAGING BIOMARKERS IN PARKINSON SPECTRUM DISORDERS

The wellspring for novel imaging biomarkers for PD and related disorders lies in the firm understanding of the pathophysiologic processes unique to these disorders based on in vitro and postmortem evaluation, which can then direct in vivo examination with PET/SPECT imaging. Recent pathologic studies have fostered a better understanding of many neurodegenerative disorders as abnormalities of protein: its increased production, abnormal folding, and/or increased deposition. Implicated proteins include α-synuclein, tau and phosphorylated tau, β-amyloid, and ubiquitin, all of which may be responsible for direct toxic effects on cells as well as activation of inflammatory microglia, loss of neuronal receptors and transporters, and changes in synaptic function or metabolism.[49–53] For example, pathologic examination of PD reveals intracellular accumulations (Lewy bodies) composed of α-synuclein, which may represent a key pathophysiologic agent in the onset and promulgation of neuronal loss.[52–54] Animal models of overexpression of α-synuclein result in a complex constellation of symptoms, which may mimic the aspects of PD. Nonetheless, there remain gaps in our mechanistic understanding of the function and pathologic role of this protein and our ability to directly image it with PET or SPECT biomarkers.

Other Parkinson spectrum disorders are characterized by overlapping but different pathology.[53] Postmortem brain examinations in PSP demonstrate loss of pigmented dopamine neurons in the substantia nigra similar to PD. However, unlike PD, there is tau protein accumulation in basal ganglia, globus pallidus, subthalamic nucleus, and substantia nigra, with formation of intracellular neurofibrillary tangles in brainstem, cortex (especially frontal lobe), dentate nucleus of cerebellum, and spinal cord. MSA demonstrates pathologic changes consistent with α-synucleinopathy, including cytoplasmic inclusions in pyramidal and extrapyramidal motor systems, cerebellar involvement, and autonomic nervous system changes; the extent and distribution of these inclusions are responsible for the major subclassification of MSA into striatonigral degeneration (mostly motor symptoms), Shy-Drager syndrome (more autonomic dysfunction in addition to motor changes), or olivopontocerebellar atrophy (with more progressive ataxia gait and dysarthria).

DLB features both intracellular α-synuclein and ubiquitin and β-amyloid deposition in extracellular plaques, whereas neurofibrillary tangles are less frequent. DLB shares the pathologic features of PD, Parkinson with dementia, and Alzheimer disease. Alzheimer disease is classically characterized by the presence of tau-containing intracellular neurofibrillary tangles and extracellular β-amyloid plaque deposits.

The importance of these advances in neuropathologic understanding of the neurodegenerative disorders lies in improving our ability to address both specific and nonspecific mechanisms for novel therapeutics and also for developing radiopharmaceuticals, which target different aspects of pathology and hence may serve as diagnostic tools or mechanistic biomarkers to monitor clinical response to a treatment intervention. This approach is in current application in several phase 3 clinical trials that are now underway of antiamyloid agents, which either disrupt the production of β-amyloid oligomers through the activity of the secretase enzyme or purport to reduce β-amyloid burden via targeted antibodies. These trials are incorporating PET imaging of amyloid burden using ^{18}F AV45 or ^{18}F florbetaben as putative mechanistic biomarkers.

The journey from identification of brain targets such as β-amyloid or α-synuclein to their incorporation into clinical algorithms or application as a biomarker in a drug trial is fraught with difficulties. Most PET or SPECT imaging agents fail during the initial human validation phases. To make the process more efficient, it is possible to set standards, which may be customized to the brain target and the proposed use. Chemical characteristics of radiotracers, which may be optimized for imaging in brain, include appropriate lipophilicity to facilitate crossing the blood brain barrier, high affinity for the target (particularly in those cases of lower target density), good signal-to-noise properties, specificity for the target of interest, and lack of metabolites, which may cross the blood brain barrier and impair quantification of the signal.[55] Other important factors include lack of P-glycoprotein substrate activity and no

significant defluorination of ^{18}F radiotracers with confounding high skull uptake. The issue of target density is particularly important for in vivo assessment of α-synuclein and other proteins, which may be in relatively low abundance. More often than not, the final assessment for the adequacy of a radiotracer must take place in early-stage human trials in which in vivo characteristics can be adequately studied, the kinetics and modeling of a quantitative outcome measure can be established, the simplified image-acquisition protocols and outcome measure can be validated, and the reproducibility of the test can be shown to be acceptable for the application for which it was designed. For example, if one has to evaluate a very slowly changing pathophysiologic process such as the accumulation of amyloid in the brain, it is important to have a good understanding of how robust, reproducible, and error-prone the imaging outcome measure must be to develop an adequate sample size for the imaging trial. In recent years, the process of radiotracer development for brain imaging has been accelerated by both the articulation of new and interesting targets as well as the establishment of the exploratory investigational new drug mechanism in the United States as a regulatory means to facilitate first-in-human studies with microdosed compounds such as radiopharmaceuticals.

Once a radiotracer has been validated for its intended use, algorithms for the incorporation of the imaging biomarker into a research application or clinical paradigms can be established. For multicenter imaging trials this presents logistic problems such as ensuring availability and distribution of radiotracer, coordinating between clinical and imaging groups at each site, and cross-site validation of PET or SPECT acquisitions across different cameras.

SUMMARY

Over the past decade, presynaptic dopaminergic SPECT and PET agents have served as clinically useful diagnostic agents (in Europe), as tools for drug development trials, and as a means for elucidating pathophysiology in vivo in cross-sectional and longitudinal studies of patients with movement disorder. From a clinical perspective, much of the work has been done in idiopathic PD, which comprises the great bulk of the parkinsonisms, and in distinguishing DLB from Alzheimer disease. Nonetheless, the limitations of presynaptic dopaminergic imaging are well understood even as more sophisticated applications of these well-used tracers remain to be established; in particular, this means pushing back the time to make the diagnosis of dopamine deficits to potentially include patients at risk for the disorder as well as patients with very early clinical signs and symptoms that do not yet meet the criteria for a diagnosis. These efforts are energized by the promise of disease-modifying drugs where the urgency for an early and accurate diagnosis becomes more acute.

As the tools for molecular imaging are expanded with new tracers, new analytic techniques for old tracers, incorporation of large-scale and well-vetted normal imaging databases, and more sophisticated clinical imaging algorithms for combining neuroimaging techniques, we should be able to make molecular diagnoses with imaging biomarkers available for smarter treatments. Hence, the applications of these biomarkers are becoming more complex across the spectrum, from detecting molecular changes in at-risk patients[27] to establishing firm differential diagnosis based on an in vivo pathology read-out to monitoring progression of disease and response to therapy on the clinical side. From a research perspective, the application of these biomarkers helps to foster smarter recruitment into clinical trials, assess mechanistic efficacy of novel treatments, and enhance understanding of pathophysiology of Parkinson spectrum disorders.

REFERENCES

1. Adler CH. Nonmotor complications in Parkinson's disease. Mov Disord 2005;20(Suppl 11):S23–9.
2. Adler CH. Differential diagnosis of Parkinson's disease. Med Clin North Am 1999;83(2):349–67.
3. Adler CH, Thorpy MJ. Sleep issues in Parkinson's disease. Neurology 2005;64(12 Suppl 3):S12–20.
4. Snyder CH, Adler CH. The patient with Parkinson's disease: part I-treating the motor symptoms; part II-treating the nonmotor symptoms. J Am Acad Nurse Pract 2007;19(4):179–97.
5. Thorpy MJ, Adler CH. Parkinson's disease and sleep. Neurol Clin 2005;23(4):1187–208.
6. Park A, Stacy M. Non-motor symptoms in Parkinson's disease. J Neurol 2009;256(Suppl 3):293–8.
7. Voon V, Fernagut PO, Wickens J, et al. Chronic dopaminergic stimulation in Parkinson's disease: from dyskinesias to impulse control disorders. Lancet Neurol 2009;8(12):1140–9.
8. Hughes AJ, Daniel SE, Blankson S, et al. A clinico-pathologic study of 100 cases of Parkinson's disease. Arch Neurol 1993;50(2):140–8.
9. Jennings DL, Seibyl JP, Oakes D, et al. (123I) beta-CIT and single-photon emission computed tomographic imaging vs clinical evaluation in Parkinsonian syndrome: unmasking an early diagnosis. Arch Neurol 2004;61(8):1224–9.
10. Seibyl J, Jennings D, Tabamo R, et al. Unique roles of SPET brain imaging in clinical and research studies. Lessons from Parkinson's disease research. Q J Nucl Med Mol Imaging 2005;49(2):215–21.
11. Tatsch K. Imaging of the dopaminergic system in differential diagnosis of dementia. Eur J Nucl Med Mol Imaging 2008;35(Suppl 1):S51–7.
12. Ravina B, Eidelberg D, Ahlskog JE, et al. The role of radiotracer imaging in Parkinson disease. Neurology 2005;64(2):208–15.
13. Seibyl J, Jennings D, Tabarno R, et al. The role of neuroimaging in the early diagnosis and evaluation of Parkinson's disease. Minerva Med 2005;96(5):353–64.
14. Dethy S, Hambye AS. [1231-FP-CIT (DaTSCAN) scintigraphy in the differential diagnosis of movement disorders]. Rev Med Brux 2008;29(4):238–47 [in French].
15. Bohnen NI, Albin RL, Koeppe RA, et al. Positron emission tomography of monoaminergic vesicular binding in aging and Parkinson disease. J Cereb Blood Flow Metab 2006;26(9):1198–212.
16. Brooks DJ, Piccini P. Imaging in Parkinson's disease: the role of monoamines in behavior. Biol Psychiatry 2006;59(10):908–18.
17. Brooks DJ. PET studies and motor complications in Parkinson's disease. Trends Neurosci 2000;23(10 Suppl):S101–8.
18. Eshuis SA, Jager PL, Maguire RP, et al. Direct comparison of FP-CIT SPECT and F-DOPA PET in patients with Parkinson's disease and healthy controls. Eur J Nucl Med Mol Imaging 2009;36(3):454–62.
19. Marek K, Jennings D, Seibyl J. Single-photon emission tomography and dopamine transporter imaging in Parkinson's disease. Adv Neurol 2003;91:183–91.
20. Marek K, Jennings D, Seibyl J. Imaging the dopamine system to assess disease-modifying drugs: studies comparing dopamine agonists and levodopa. Neurology 2003;61(6 Suppl 3):S43–8.
21. Marek K, Jennings D, Tamagnan G, et al. Biomarkers for Parkinson's [corrected] disease: tools to assess Parkinson's disease onset and progression. Ann Neurol 2008;64(Suppl 2):S111–21.
22. Varrone A, Marek KL, Jennings D, et al. [(123)I]beta-CIT SPECT imaging demonstrates reduced density of striatal dopamine transporters in Parkinson's disease and multiple system atrophy. Mov Disord 2001;16(6):1023–32.
23. Volonte MA, Moresco RM, Gobbo C, et al. A PET study with [11-C]raclopride in Parkinson's disease: preliminary results on the effect of amantadine on the dopaminergic system. Neurol Sci 2001;22(1):107–8.
24. de la Fuente-Fernandez R, Stoessl AJ. Parkinson's disease: imaging update. Curr Opin Neurol 2002;15(4):477–82.
25. de la Fuente-Fernandez R, Sossi V, Huang Z, et al. Levodopa-induced changes in synaptic dopamine

levels increase with progression of Parkinson's disease: implications for dyskinesias. Brain 2004; 127(Pt 12):2747–54.

26. Linazasoro G, Antonini A, Maguire RP, et al. Pharmacological and PET studies in patient's with Parkinson's disease and a short duration-motor response: implications in the pathophysiology of motor complications. J Neural Transm 2004;111(4):497–509.

27. Marek K, Jennings D. Can we image premotor Parkinson disease? Neurology 2009;72(7 Suppl):S21–6.

28. Juh R, Kim J, Moon D, et al. Different metabolic patterns analysis of Parkinsonism on the 18F-FDG PET. Eur J Radiol 2004;51(3):223–33.

29. Poston KL, Eidelberg D. Network biomarkers for the diagnosis and treatment of movement disorders. Neurobiol Dis 2009;35(2):141–7.

30. Ma Y, Huang C, Dyke JP, et al. Parkinson's disease spatial covariance pattern: noninvasive quantification with perfusion MRI. J Cereb Blood Flow Metab 2010;30(3):505–9.

31. Huang C, Mattis P, Perrine K, et al. Metabolic abnormalities associated with mild cognitive impairment in Parkinson disease. Neurology 2008;70(16 Pt 2): 1470–7.

32. Huang C, Tang C, Feigin A, et al. Changes in network activity with the progression of Parkinson's disease. Brain 2007;130(Pt 7):1834–46.

33. Spetsieris PG, Ma Y, Dhawan V, et al. Differential diagnosis of parkinsonian syndromes using PCA-based functional imaging features. Neuroimage 2009;45(4):1241–52.

34. Nakajima K, Yoshita M, Matsuo S, et al. Iodine-123-MIBG sympathetic imaging in Lewy-body diseases and related movement disorders. Q J Nucl Med Mol Imaging 2008;52(4):378–87.

35. Oka H, Yoshioka M, Morita M, et al. Reduced cardiac 123I-MIBG uptake reflects cardiac sympathetic dysfunction in Lewy body disease. Neurology 2007;69(14):1460–5.

36. Post KK, Singer C, Papapetropoulos S. Cardiac denervation and dysautonomia in Parkinson's disease: a review of screening techniques. Parkinsonism Relat Disord 2008;14(7):524–31.

37. Spiegel J, Mollers MO, Jost WH, et al. FP-CIT and MIBG scintigraphy in early Parkinson's disease. Mov Disord 2005;20(5):552–61.

38. Sawada H, Oeda T, Yamamoto K, et al. Diagnostic accuracy of cardiac metaiodobenzylguanidine scintigraphy in Parkinson disease. Eur J Neurol 2009;16(2): 174–82.

39. Chauveau F, Boutin H, Van Camp N, et al. Nuclear imaging of neuroinflammation: a comprehensive review of [11C]PK11195 challengers. Eur J Nucl Med Mol Imaging 2008;35(12):2304–19.

40. Dolle F, Luus C, Reynolds A, et al. Radiolabelled molecules for imaging the translocator protein (18 kDa) using positron emission tomography. Curr Med Chem 2009;16(22):2899–923.

41. Chen MK, Guilarte TR. Translocator protein 18 kDa (TSPO): molecular sensor of brain injury and repair. Pharmacol Ther 2008;118(1):1–17.

42. Gerhard A, Pavese N, Hotton G, et al. In vivo imaging of microglial activation with [11C](R)-PK11195 PET in idiopathic Parkinson's disease. Neurobiol Dis 2006;21(2):404–12.

43. Gerhard A, Trender-Gerhard I, Turkheimer F, et al. In vivo imaging of microglial activation with [11C](R)-PK11195 PET in progressive supranuclear palsy. Mov Disord 2006;21(1):89–93.

44. Menke RA, Scholz J, Miller KL, et al. MRI characteristics of the substantia nigra in Parkinson's disease: a combined quantitative T1 and DTI study. Neuroimage 2009;47(2):435–41.

45. Gattellaro G, Minati L, Grisoli M, et al. White matter involvement in idiopathic Parkinson disease: a diffusion tensor imaging study. AJNR Am J Neuroradiol 2009;30(6):1222–6.

46. Vaillancourt DE, Spraker MB, Prodoehl J, et al. High-resolution diffusion tensor imaging in the substantia nigra of de novo Parkinson disease. Neurology 2009;72(16):1378–84.

47. Tessa C, Giannelli M, Della Nave R, et al. A whole-brain analysis in de novo Parkinson disease. AJNR Am J Neuroradiol 2008;29(4):674–80.

48. Chan LL, Rumpel H, Yap K, et al. Case control study of diffusion tensor imaging in Parkinson's disease. J Neurol Neurosurg Psychiatry 2007;78(12):1383–6.

49. Singleton AB, Farrer M, Johnson J, et al. alpha-Synuclein locus triplication causes Parkinson's disease. Science 2003;302(5646):841.

50. Braak H, Del Tredici K, Rub U, et al. Staging of brain pathology related to sporadic Parkinson's disease. Neurobiol Aging 2003;24(2):197–211.

51. Murray B, Lynch T, Farrell M. Clinicopathological features of the tauopathies. Biochem Soc Trans 2005;33(Pt 4):595–9.

52. Kao AW, Racine CA, Quitania LC, et al. Cognitive and neuropsychiatric profile of the synucleinopathies: Parkinson disease, dementia with lewy bodies, and multiple system atrophy. Alzheimer Dis Assoc Disord 2009;23(4):365–70.

53. Tong J, Wong H, Guttman M, et al. Brain alpha-synuclein accumulation in multiple system atrophy, Parkinson's disease and progressive supranuclear palsy: a comparative investigation. Brain 2010;133(Pt 1):172–88.

54. O'Keeffe GC, Michell AW, Barker RA. Biomarkers in Huntington's and Parkinson's disease. Ann N Y Acad Sci 2009;1180:97–110.

55. Guilloteau D, Chalon S. PET and SPECT exploration of central monoaminergic transporters for the development of new drugs and treatments in brain disorders. Curr Pharm Des 2005;11(25):3237–45.

^{18}F-AV-133: A Selective VMAT2-binding Radiopharmaceutical for PET Imaging of Dopaminergic Neurons

Franz F. Hefti, PhD[a], Hank F. Kung, PhD[b],
Michael R. Kilbourn, PhD[c], Alan P. Carpenter, PhD, JD[a],
Christopher M. Clark, MD[a,b,d],
Daniel M. Skovronsky, MD, PhD[a,b],*

KEYWORDS

- ^{18}F-AV-133 • Dopaminergic neurons • Imaging agents
- PET imaging

The early detection and monitoring of neurodegenerative diseases, including Parkinson disease (PD), Alzheimer disease (AD), dementia with Lewy bodies (DLB) and other dementias, and movement disorders, represent a significant unmet medical need. Disease mechanisms are gradually becoming understood, and disease-modifying drugs that target the specific molecular pathology underlying each of these diseases are emerging. Tools for accurate and early differential diagnosis are thus necessary to determine the appropriate treatment for patients and to minimize inappropriate use of potentially harmful treatments. In addition, such diagnostic imaging tools are expected to permit monitoring of disease progression and will thus accelerate testing and development of disease-modifying drugs. Furthermore, the new imaging tests may be useful as prognostic tools by identifying humans with neurodegenerative diseases before the clinical manifestations become evident.

Most of the motor deficits that represent the cardinal symptoms of PD are caused by the progressive degeneration of dopaminergic neurons of the midbrain, which project to the basal ganglia of the forebrain and synaptically release the transmitter dopamine (DA) on target neurons there. The midbrain dopaminergic neuronal population also undergoes degeneration in patients with DLB, thereby generating parkinsonian symptoms. Given the essential role of DA neurons in these diseases, the development of suitable imaging tools has been an active research endeavor in recent years.

APPROACHES TO DA NEURON IMAGING

The 3 types of imaging agents that have been developed so far are (1) agents imaging the enzymatic activity of aromatic amino acid decarboxylase (AADC), which converts L-dihydroxyphenylalanine (L-DOPA) to DA; (2) agents imaging the dopamine transporters (DAT) that are located at the extracellular membrane and responsible for the reuptake of DA from the synaptic cleft, and (3) agents imaging vesicular monoamine transporter type 2 (VMAT2) located on the membranes

[a] Avid Radiopharmaceuticals Inc, 3711 Market Street, 7th Floor, Philadelphia, PA 19104, USA
[b] Department of Radiology, University of Pennsylvania, Philadelphia, PA 19104, USA
[c] Department of Radiology, University of Michigan, Ann Arbor, MI, USA
[d] Department of Neurology, University of Pennsylvania, Philadelphia, PA 19104, USA
* Corresponding author. Avid Radiopharmaceuticals Inc, 3711 Market Street, 7th Floor, Philadelphia, PA 19104.
E-mail address: skrovronsky@avidrp.com

PET Clin 5 (2010) 75–82
doi:10.1016/j.cpet.2010.02.001
1556-8598/10/$ – see front matter © 2010 Published by Elsevier Inc.

of the intracellular vesicles storing DA for synaptic release.

[18F]6-Fluoro-DOPA

[18F]6-Fluoro-DOPA (FDOPA) is the PET imaging agent for dopaminergic neuron function and it is a commonly used PET agent. FDOPA is a false substrate for the enzyme AADC. PET imaging with [18F]6-FDOPA reflects the in situ synthesis of DA.[1,2] Because AADC is not only localized in dopaminergic neurons and AADC enzyme appears to be up-regulated in the parkinsonian brain, and because the O-methylated derivatives are contributing to background noise, [18F]6-FDO-PA imaging may underestimate the degree of neuronal loss caused by compensatory changes.[3–5]

DAT Ligands

Several ligands for DAT, which is responsible for the reuptake of DA from the synaptic cleft, have been pursued as radiopharmaceuticals. These ligands include iodine-123-fluoropropyl-β-carbo-methoxy-3β-(4-iodophenyltropane) (123I-FP-CIT, DaTSCAN), which has been approved as a single photon emission computed tomography (SPECT) radiopharmaceutical. Most of the DAT imaging agents are tropane (or cocaine) derivatives, which have varying degrees of affinity to serotonin and norepinephrine transporters.[6–13] These agents are likely to be superior to FDOPA as imaging agents. A review by Ravina and colleagues[14] pointed out the deficiencies in imaging

dopaminergic neuron function based on DAT tracers. There is evidence from animals suggesting that DA agonist therapy, given to most patients with PD, may affect the expression of DAT, and thus limit their utility to accurately reflect the structural integrity of dopaminergic systems. The currently broadly available DAT SPECT radiopharmaceuticals provide images of lower spatial resolution than is possible with 18F-PET. Quantization of dopaminergic neuronal changes over time is also anticipated to be better with 18F agents because of the inherent higher image resolution achievable with PET compared with SPECT.

VMAT2 Ligands

The third type of imaging agent for dopaminergic neurons is VMAT2-specific tracers. 11C-labeled tetrabenazine (TBZ) derivatives, including [11C]di-hydrotetrabenazine ([11C]DTBZ), have been successfully tested in humans. An 18F-labeled agent, [18F]9-fluoropropyl-DTBZ (18F-AV-133) is in early stages of clinical development as a commercial radiopharmaceutical. These VMAT2-specific tracer molecules are discussed in detail in the following sections.

VMAT2 AS PET IMAGING TARGET

VMAT2 is an integral part of the mechanism for vesicular packaging and storage of monoamine neurotransmitters in the synapses of the brain (**Fig. 1**, see Refs.[15–19] for reviews). After synthesis of monoamines in the presynaptic terminals, the

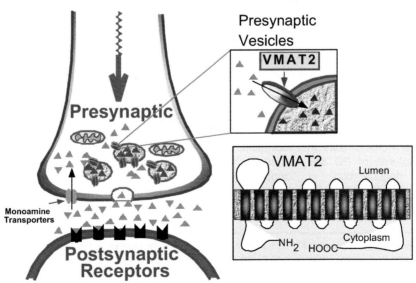

Fig. 1. VMAT2, the molecular target of 11C-DTBZ and 18F-AV-133. Schematic drawing of a typical monoamine neuron (*left*). VMAT2s are located in the presynaptic neurons that are responsible for storing and packing the neurotransmitters (*small triangles*) inside the vesicles. VMAT2 is a 12-domain transmembrane protein that selectively transports monoamines (DA, serotonin, norepinephrine) into transmitter storage vesicles.

transmitter molecules are transported into the vesicles by VMAT2. This transporter does not differentiate among monoamines and is responsible for the movement of dopamine, norepinephrine, and serotonin from the cytosol into the vesicles, providing a potential utility as imaging agent for all monoaminergic neurons in the brain. The selectivity of the vesicular transporter VMAT2 is different from that of monoamine transporters on the synaptic membrane, where there are specific and distinct transporters for active reuptake of 3 monoamines (DAT, norepinephrine transporter, and serotonin transporter). VMAT2 is an ATP-dependent transporter, related to VMAT1, the catecholamine transporter expressed in adrenal cells. In the brain, the expression of VMAT2 is highly restricted to the monoaminergic neurons. Outside the central nervous system, VMAT2 expression has also been established for the pancreas, thus providing a further potential utility as imaging agent for diabetes as discussed later.

VMAT2 is inhibited by reserpine and TBZ, which bind to the transporter with high affinity. By inhibiting VMAT2, reserpine and TBZ shunt most of the synthesized monoamine directly toward metabolism, therefore acting as monoamine depleting agents and inhibiting monoaminergic neurotransmission. Reserpine was used medically as an antipsychotic drug and sedative but has been replaced by more specific drugs in the recent past. TBZ has been approved in several countries for the treatment of hyperkinetic movement disorders. Several reports[20,21] have been published regarding the safety and adverse effects from the short- and long-term use of TBZ. The most commonly reported side effects included drowsiness, parkinsonism, depression, and akathisia. The chemical structure of TBZ has served as the starting point to generate useful VMAT2 PET imaging agents.

[11C]Dihydrotetrabenazine

The first useful VMAT2 imaging agent synthesized was [11C]DTBZ. Because TBZ was known to be rapidly reduced in vivo to the corresponding hydroxyl compound DTBZ,[22] radioligand development for PET imaging focused on the synthesis of [11C]DTBZ itself.[23] Racemic [11C](±)-DTBZ consists of at least 2 enantiomers, of which, [11C](+)-DTBZ is the active isomer.[23,24] Synthesis of the single optically resolved isomer [11C](+)-DTBZ (labeled at the 9-MeO position) provided the most specific PET tracer for measuring VMAT2 sites in the brain.[23]

[11C]DTBZ has been successfully tested in humans.[3] More than 50 patients received

[11C](±)-DTBZ and more than 150 patients received [11C](+)-DTBZ.[4,25–29] The imaging agents were found to be safe and useful as diagnostic imaging agents in humans to visualize the terminal areas of dopaminergic neurons in the basal ganglia.

Data from animals suggest that [11C]DTBZ is not sensitive to drugs affecting DA levels in the brain, providing an advantage over DAT imaging agents. Binding of VMAT2 ligands are therefore believed to most accurately reflect the structural integrity of monoamine neurons.[3,27,30,31]

The short half-life (20 minutes) of the imaging agents labeled with ^{11}C has precluded widespread use and commercialization. We have developed an ^{18}F-labeled VMAT2 imaging agent that has a half-life of 110 minutes and can be used more easily and more widely.

18F-AV-133: a Selective PET Radiopharmaceutical for VMAT2

Given the advantages of ^{18}F-labeled radiopharmaceuticals, we have developed ^{18}F-AV-133, the first ^{18}F-labeled VMAT2 imaging agent that has entered clinical trials.[23,32,33] ^{18}F-AV-133 is structurally similar but not identical to [11C]DTBZ, which in turn is a derivative of TBZ. Fig. 2 shows the structural relationship between ^{18}F-AV-133 and TBZ.

^{18}F-AV-133 has been characterized in detail in pharmacological studies in rats.[33] Briefly, the compound binds to homogenates of rat brain tissue from the corpus striatum, the terminal area of DA neurons, with a high affinity ($K_i = 0.10$ nM). When administered intravenously to mice, ^{18}F-AV-133 shows good penetration into and rapid clearance from the brain. Concentrations of ^{18}F-AV-133 in the brain reach 3.5% dose/g within 2 minutes after administration and decrease to 1.0% dose/g within 60 minutes. Localization of the tracer in the brain examined by ex vivo autoradiography displayed a distribution pattern consistent with VMAT2 sites. The selective labeling of the tracer in the dopaminergic neuron terminal area (corpus striatum) was almost completely abolished in animals in which the dopaminergic neurons had been destroyed by injections of 6-hydroxydopamine.

^{18}F-AV-133 binding to VMAT2 is highly selective because the compound does not show significant binding to a large battery of other G protein-coupled receptors and functionally relevant ion channels. The potential toxicity of unlabeled compound was tested in rats and dogs with single acute and repeated doses. No adverse effects were observed in these studies up to the highest doses tested, which corresponded to 50 times

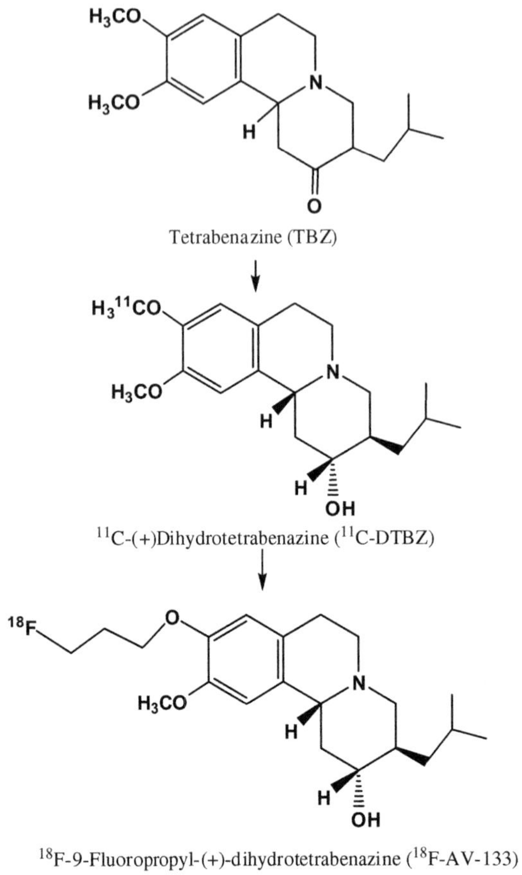

Tetrabenazine (TBZ)

^{11}C-(+)Dihydrotetrabenazine (^{11}C-DTBZ)

^{18}F-9-Fluoropropyl-(+)-dihydrotetrabenazine (^{18}F-AV-133)

Fig. 2. Structural relationship of ^{18}F-AV-133 to TBZ and DTBZ. In ^{18}F-AV-133, a propyl linker has been added to attach the ^{18}F label without altering the core structure and preserving the stereochemistry of DTBZ.

the maximal intended human dose. Potential genetic toxicity was tested using the standard in vitro and in vivo assays. The compound was negative at all doses and in all models tested, indicating minimal risk of genotoxicity.

^{18}F-AV-133 was further evaluated in a PET imaging study in rhesus monkeys. The compound showed rapid uptake into the brain with the maximum signal within 2 minutes after injection followed by rapid washout. The basal ganglia, which are rich in dopaminergic terminals, were visualized distinctively by PET imaging (**Fig. 3**). A further study was done to show that binding of ^{18}F-AV-133 to VMAT2 in the primate brain was reversible and could be competed for by a large dose of cold TBZ. The findings indicate that ^{18}F-AV-133 readily enters the primate brain and localizes in the expected VMAT2-rich region.[32] The imaging studies in monkeys indicate that ^{18}F-AV-133 is highly useful as a PET imaging agent and

that it visualizes VMAT2-binding sites in a highly selective way.

^{18}F-AV-133 in the Diagnosis of Neurodegenerative Diseases

^{18}F-AV-133 is currently being studied in clinical trials with patients suffering from movement disorders or dementia. In movement disorders, a VMAT2-imaging agent may be useful in the diagnosis of PD and its differentiation from other movement disorders. The clinical differential diagnosis of PD includes essential tremor, vascular parkinsonism, progressive supranuclear palsy, and various forms of drug-induced parkinsonism, conditions that are typically not associated with profound degeneration of DA neurons like PD.[34–36] In addition, a VMAT2 imaging agent may be useful in monitoring the progression of PD in trials with disease-modifying drugs. Recent examples of such studies include testing of glial cell-derived neurotrophic factor, in which imaging of DA neurons with FDOPA yielded conflicting results, resulting in the wide recognition of the need for better imaging agents for DA neurons.

In the clinical area of dementia, VMAT2 imaging agents may be useful in the diagnosis of DLB and its differentiation from other dementias. The prevalence of DLB is estimated to be 15% to 30% of all cases of dementia.[37,38] Given the difficulty in diagnosing DLB in living patients and the fact the AD is often used as default diagnosis of dementia, it is possible that the actual prevalence is yet higher. The behavioral symptoms of DLB, in addition to dementia, include fluctuations in activity and alertness, nonthreatening hallucinations, and parkinsonian hypokinesia.[39–44] In contrast to AD, the behavioral changes tend to be less stable than those of AD and to vary often during relatively short time intervals. The DLB postmortem pathology includes Lewy bodies in subcortical and cortical regions, degenerative changes of the dopaminergic systems, as well as Aβ aggregates.[40–43,45] The pathological changes are clearly distinct from those of AD, which include abundant deposits of neurofibrillary tangles and no significant degenerative changes of the dopaminergic systems. The pathological changes of DLB are quantitatively and qualitatively distinct from those of PD, which is characterized by almost complete degeneration of dopaminergic systems, Lewy body abundance in midbrain structure, and little Aβ aggregate pathology. Imaging the dopaminergic neurons with the SPECT radiopharmaceutical, DaTSCAN, was found to substantially enhance the accuracy of diagnosis of DLB compared with clinical criteria alone.[46]

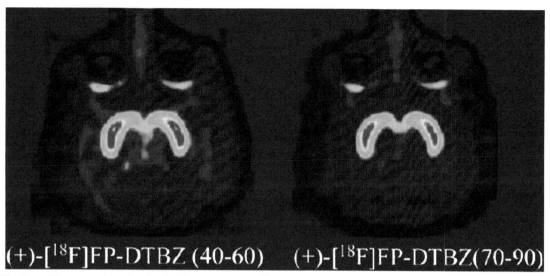

(+)-[18F]FP-DTBZ (40-60)   (+)-[18F]FP-DTBZ(70-90)

Fig. 3. PET images of monkey brain after injection of 18F-AV-133. The high uptake and localization in the VMAT2 region (striatum) is clearly evident.

Hypersensitivity to neuroleptics is a key feature of patients with DLB. Approximately 50% of the patients with DLB and none of the patients with AD showed severe reactions to neuroleptics in a controlled study.[40–43,47,48] These reactions included increased parkinsonian motor dysfunction and cognitive worsening. The hypersensitivity to neuroleptics is thought to reflect dopamine receptor hypersensitivity in response to dopaminergic neuron degeneration. Neuroleptic sensitivity can cause significant adverse events in patients, making it important to avoid exposure of potentially vulnerable patients.

An international consortium has established guidelines for the behavioral and pathologic diagnosis of DLB.[40–43] The consortium emphasized the utility of imaging techniques for the diagnosis, in particular the differential diagnosis from AD.[40–43]

Use of 18F-AV-133 Beyond DA Neuron Imaging

VMAT2 is expressed by dopaminergic, noradrenergic, and serotonergic neurons in the brain, and therefore provides an opportunity to gain imaging information beyond the target area of the dopaminergic neurons. Norepinephrine is the transmitter of an important modulatory neural system, the ascending noradrenergic pathway, emanating from the locus coeruleus. The neurons project to essentially all brain areas, making the system one of the dominant, divergent, modulatory systems of the brain. Similarly, the serotonergic neurons form a divergent modulatory system. Their cell bodies are localized in several brainstem nuclei from which distinct ascending and descending pathways emerge. Most important are the ascending pathways that originate in the dorsal and medial raphe nuclei and innervate most of the forebrain areas. Noradrenergic and serotonergic neurons are thought to play a significant role in depression, because the currently approved antidepressant drugs target receptor sites of monoaminergic transmitter molecules and they are likely to be involved in aspects of mood in normal and pathological conditions.

In contrast to the dopaminergic neurons of the mesencephalon, which provide a very dense innervation to well circumscribed target areas that are highly visible in VMAT2 PET imaging, the diffuse innervation provided by noradrenergic and serotonergic neurons may make precise quantification more difficult. However, their cell bodies, which are densely packed in small nuclei, may provide a target for PET imaging. PET signal intensity in the cell body areas may provide a reflection of the structural integrity of these systems.

In addition to the obvious utility of VMAT2 imaging agents for imaging monoaminergic neurons in the brain in neurological disorders, there may be a surprising additional utility in diabetes. Immunohistochemical staining studies of gene expression in the endocrine pancreas showed that VMAT2-binding sites are expressed mainly on the β-cells of the pancreas.[49,50] VMAT2 expression also correlates well with the insulin levels in the pancreas of humans and monkeys.[51] Therefore, VMAT2 may be an excellent target for following changes in pancreatic β-cell mass.

The early detection and monitoring of pancreatic β-cell mass in type 1 and type 2 diabetes represents a significant unmet medical need. Disease mechanisms are fairly well understood, and novel disease-modifying drugs that target specific molecular pathology underlying diabetes are emerging. Tools for accurate and early differential diagnosis are thus necessary to determine the appropriate treatment for patients and to minimize inappropriate use of potentially harmful treatments. In addition, such diagnostic imaging tools are expected to permit monitoring of disease progression and will thus accelerate testing and development of disease-modifying drugs. Furthermore, the new imaging test may be useful as prognostic tools by identifying humans suffering from diabetes before the clinical manifestations become evident. So far, attempts have been made to image β-cell mass based on specific binding sites in the pancreas (ie, sulfonylurea receptors and other binding sites.[52–54] Studies using β-cell–specific antibody and fragments as in vivo imaging agents have shown some utility but are not suitable for routine clinical use because of low pancreatic cellular specificity.[55] Imaging agents for VMAT2 thus warrant further investigations on their clinical utility for imaging β-cell mass in the pancreas. ^{18}F-AV-133 is currently in exploratory clinical studies in this patient population.

REFERENCES

1. Brooks DJ. The early diagnosis of Parkinson's disease. Ann Neurol 1998;44:S10.
2. Whone AL, Bailey DL, Remy P, et al. A technique for standardized central analysis of 6-(18)F-fluoro-L-DOPA PET data from a multicenter study. J Nucl Med 2004;45:1135–45.
3. Frey KA, Koeppe RA, Kilbourn MR, et al. Imaging the vesicular monoamine transporter. Adv Neurol 2001;86:237.
4. Lee CS, Samii A, Sossi V, et al. In vivo positron emission tomographic evidence for compensatory changes in presynaptic dopaminergic nerve terminals in Parkinson's disease. Ann Neurol 2000;47:493.
5. Tatsch K. Can SPET imaging of dopamine uptake sites replace PET imaging in Parkinson's disease? Eur J Nucl Med Mol Imaging 2002;29:711.
6. Booij J, Tissingh G, Winogrodzka A, et al. Imaging of the dopaminergic neurotransmission system using single-photon emission tomography and positron emission tomography in patients with parkinsonism. Eur J Nucl Med 1999;26:171.
7. Booij J, Speelman JD, Horstink MW, et al. The clinical benefit of imaging striatal dopamine transporters with [123I]FP-CIT SPET in differentiating patients with presynaptic parkinsonism from those with other forms of parkinsonism. Eur J Nucl Med 2001;28:266.
8. Ding YS, Fowler JS, Volkow ND, et al. Carbon-11-d-threo-methylphenidate binding to dopamine transporter in baboon brain. J Nucl Med 1995;36:2298.
9. Innis RB. Single photon emission computed tomography imaging of dopaminergic function: presynaptic transporter, postsynaptic receptor, and "intrasynaptic" transmitter. Adv Pharmacol 1998; 42:215.
10. Meegalla SK, Ploëssl K, Kung MP, et al. Specificity of diastereomers of [99mTc]TRODAT-1 as dopamine transporter imaging agents. J Med Chem 1998;41:428.
11. Mozley PD, Schneider JS, Acton PD, et al. Binding of [99mTc]TRODAT-1 to dopamine transporters in patients with Parkinson's disease and in healthy volunteers. J Nucl Med 2000;41:584.
12. Volkow ND, Ding YS, Fowler JS, et al. Dopamine transporters decrease with age. J Nucl Med 1996; 37:554.
13. Volkow ND, Fowler JS, Gatley SJ, et al. PET evaluation of the dopamine system of the human brain. J Nucl Med 1996;37:1242.
14. Ravina BD, Eidelberg JE, Ahlskog JE, et al. The role of radiotracer imaging in Parkinson disease. Neurology 2005;64:208.
15. Yelin R, Schuldiner S. Vesicular neurotransmitter transporters: pharmacology, biochemistry, and molecular analysis. In: Reith MEA, editor. Neurotransmitter transporters; structure, function, and regulation. 2nd edition. Totowa (NJ): Humana Press; 2002. p. 313–54.
16. Zhang W, Oya S, Kung MP, et al. F-18 stilbenes as PET imaging agents for detecting beta-amyloid plaques in the brain. J Med Chem 2005;48:5980–8.
17. Zhang W, Oya S, Kung MP, et al. F-18 polyethelene-glycol stilbenes as PET imaging agents for detecting Abeta aggregates in the brain. Nucl Med Biol 2005; 32:799–809.
18. Zhang W, Kung MP, Oya S, et al. 18F-labeled styryl-pyridines as PET agents for amyloid plaque imaging. Nucl Med Biol 2007;34:89–97.
19. Zheng G, Dwoskin LP, Crooks PA. Vesicular monoamine transporter 2: role as a novel target for drug development. AAPS J 2006;28:E682–92.
20. Kenney C, Hunter C, Jankovic J. Long-term tolerability of tetrabenazine in the treatment of hyperkinetic movement disorders. Mov Disord 2007;22:193–7.
21. Jankovic J, Beach J. Long-term effects of tetrabenazine in hyperkinetic movement disorders. Neurology 1997;48:358–62.
22. Mehvar R, Jamali F, Watson MW, et al. Pharmacokinetics of tetrabenazine and its major metabolite in

man and rat. Bioavailability and dose dependency studies. Drug Metab Dispos 1987;15:250–1.

23. Kilbourn MR, Lee LC, Heeg MJ, et al. Absolute configuration of (1)alphadihydrotetrabenazine, an active metabolite of tetrabenazine. Chirality 1997;9: 59–62.

24. Kilbourn M, Sherman P. In vivo binding of (1)-[alpha]-[3H]dihydrotetrabenazine to the vesicular monoamine transporter of rat brain: bolus vs. equilibrium studies. Eur J Pharmacol 1997b;331:161–8.

25. Adams JR, van Netten H, Schulzer M, et al. PET in LRRK2 mutations: comparison to sporadic Parkinson's disease and evidence for presymptomatic compensation. Brain 2005;128:2777–85.

26. Albin RL, Koeppe RA, Chervin RD, et al. Decreased striatal dopaminergic innervation in REM sleep behavior disorder. Neurology 2000;55: 1410–2.

27. Bohnen NI, Albin RL, Koeppe RA, et al. Positron emission tomography of monoaminergic vesicular binding in aging and Parkinson disease. J Cereb Blood Flow Metab 2006;9:1198–212.

28. Koeppe RA, Gilman S, Joshi A, et al. 11C-DTBZ and 18F-FDG PET measures in differentiating dementias. J Nucl Med 2005;46:936–44.

29. Kumar A, Mann S, Sossi V, et al. [11C]DTBZ-PET correlates of levodopa responses in asymmetric Parkinson's disease. Brain 2003;126:2648–55.

30. Kilbourn MR, Frey KA, Vander Borght T, et al. Effects of dopaminergic drug treatments on in vivo radioligand binding to brain vesicular monoamine transporters. Nucl Med Biol 1996;23:467.

31. Lee CS, Schulzer M, de la Fuente-Fernandez R, et al. Lack of regional selectivity during the progression of Parkinson disease: implications for pathogenesis. Arch Neurol 1920;61:2004.

32. Kilbourn MR, Hockley B, Lee L, et al. Pharmacokinetics of [18F]fluoroalkyl derivatives of dihydrotetrabenazine (DTBZ) in rat and monkey brain. Nucl Med Biol 2007;34:233–7.

33. Kung MP, Hou C, Goswami R, et al. Characterization of optically resolved 9-fluoropropyldihydrotetrabenazine as a potential PET imaging agent targeting vesicular monoamine transporters. Nucl Med Biol 2007;34:239–46.

34. Fahn S. Description of Parkinson's disease as a clinical syndrome. Ann N Y Acad Sci 2003;991:1–14.

35. Gilman S. Parkinsonian syndromes. Clin Geriatr Med 2006;22:827–42.

36. Tolosa E, Wenning G, Poewe W. The diagnosis of Parkinson's disease. Lancet Neurol 2006;5:75–86.

37. Holmes C, Cairns N, Lantos P, et al. Validity of current clinical criteria for Alzheimer disease, vascular dementia and dementia with Lewy bodies. Br J Psychol 1999;174:45–50.

38. Luis CA, Mittenberg W, Gass CS, et al. Diffuse Lewy body disease: clinical, pathological, and neuropsychological review. Neuropsychol Rev 1999;9:139–50.

39. Geldmacher DS. Dementia with Lewy bodies: diagnosis and clinical approach. Cleve Clin J Med 2004;71:789–99.

40. McKeith IG, Galalsko D, Kosaka K, et al. Consensus guidelines for the clinical and pathologic diagnosis of dementia with Lewy bodies (DLB): report of the consortium on DLB international workshop. Neurology 1996;47:1113–24.

41. McKeith IG, Perry EK, Perry RH, et al. Report of the second dementia with Lewy body international workshop. Neurology 1999;53:902–5.

42. McKeith IG. Dementia with Lewy bodies. Br J Psychol 2002;180:144–7.

43. McKeith IG, Dickson DW, Lowe J, et al. Diagnosis and management of dementia with Lewy bodies: third report of the DLB consortium. Neurology 2005;65:1863–72.

44. Stavitsky K, Brickman AM, Scarmeas N, et al. The progression of cognition, psychiatric symptoms, and functional abilities in dementia with Lewy bodies and Alzheimer's disease. Arch Neurol 2006;63: 1450–65.

45. Deramecourt V, Bombois S, Maurage CA, et al. Biochemical staging of synuclineopathy and amyloid deposition in dementia with Lewy bodies. J Neuropathol Exp Neurol 2006;65:278–88.

46. Walker Z, Jaros E, Walker RW, et al. Dementia with Lewy bodies: a comparison of clinical diagnosis, FP-CIT single photon emission computed tomography imaging and autopsy. J Neurol Neurosurg Psychiatry 2007;78:1176–81.

47. Aarsland D, Perry R, Larsen JP, et al. Neuroleptic sensitivity in Parkinson disease and parkinsonian dementias. J Clin Psychiatry 2005;66:633–7.

48. Baskys A. Lewy body dementia: the litmus test for neuroleptic sensitivity and extrapyramidal symptoms. J Clin Psychiatry 2004;65(Suppl 11):16–22.

49. Harris PE, Ferrara C, Barba P, et al. VMAT2 gene expression and function as it applies to imaging beta-cell mass. J Mol Med 2008;86:5–16.

50. Maffei A, Liu Z, Witkowski P, et al. Identification of tissue-restricted transcripts in human islets. Endocrinology 2004;145:4513–21.

51. Anlauf M, Eissele R, Schafer MK, et al. Expression of the two isoforms of the vesicular monoamine transporter (VMAT 1 and VMAT 2) in the endocrine pancreas and pancreatic endocrine tumors. J Histochem Cytochem 2003;51:1027–40.

52. Schmitz A, Shiue CY, Feng Q, et al. Synthesis and evaluation of fluorine-18 labeled glyburide analogs as beta-cell imaging agents. Nucl Med Biol 2004; 31:483–91.

53. Wangler B, Schneider S, Thews O, et al. Synthesis and evaluation of (S)-2-(2-[18F]fluoroethoxy)-4-([3-methyl-1-(2-piperidin-1-yl-phenyl)-butyl-carbamoyl]-

methyl)-benzoic acid ([18F]repaglinide): a promising radioligand for quantification of pancreatic betacell mass with positron emission tomography (PET). Nucl Med Biol 2004;31:639–47.

54. Clark PB, Gage HD, Brown-Proctor C, et al. Neurofunctional imaging of the pancreas utilizing the cholinergic PET radioligand [18F]4-fluorobenzyltrozamicol. Eur J Nucl Med Mol Imaging 2004;31:258–60.

55. Hampe CS, Wallen AR, Schlosser M, et al. Quantitative evaluation of a monoclonal antibody and its fragment as potential markers for pancreatic beta cell mass. Exp Clin Endocrinol Diabetes 2005;113: 381–7.

PET in Cerebrovascular Disease

William J. Powers, MD[a],*, Allyson R. Zazulia, MD[b,c]

KEYWORDS

- Positron emission tomography
- Cerebrovascular disease • Vascular dementia
- Cerebral blood flow • Cerebral metabolism
- Cerebral hemodynamics

Cerebrovascular disease results from a derangement of the normal relationship between the cerebral vasculature and the brain parenchyma. Thus, investigation of the interplay between the cerebral circulation and brain cellular function is fundamental to understanding both the pathophysiology and treatment of stroke. At present, PET is the only technique that provides accurate, quantitative in vivo regional measurements of both cerebral circulation and cellular metabolism in human subjects. PET is therefore well suited for the study of human cerebrovascular disease, but its application to this end is not easy. An on-site cyclotron and radiochemistry facility is necessary due to the short half-lives of the commonly used radionuclides [15]O (2 minutes) and [11]C (20 minutes). Quantitative physiologic measurements require complex post-processing and multiple arterial blood samples, although for some specific applications simple count-based images can be used.[1,2] Patients with acute stroke may be medically unstable, requiring a nurse or physician in attendance. For these reasons, PET is still a research tool for cerebrovascular disease. PET has provided us with valuable new knowledge and insight into both ischemic and hemorrhagic stroke regarding pathophysiology, therapy, and prognosis but has not entered the mainstream of clinical practice. In the future, the results of the Carotid Occlusion Surgery Study (www.cosstrial.org), an ongoing clinical trial in which PET is being used to determine eligibility, may demonstrate the clinical value of PET for the routine management of cerebrovascular disease.

NORMAL CEREBRAL HEMODYNAMICS AND ENERGY METABOLISM

Energy in the brain is used for the maintenance of membrane potentials, for the biosynthesis and transport of neurotransmitters, and for the biosynthesis and transport of cellular elements. Under normal circumstances the brain relies on a continuous supply of oxygen and glucose from the blood for its functional and structural integrity.[3] Because storage of substrates for energy metabolism in the brain is minimal, it is exquisitely sensitive to even brief disturbances in this supply. Complete interruption of the cerebral circulation in cardiac arrest causes loss of consciousness within 10 seconds.[4]

This work was supported by USPHS grants NS06833, NS35966, NS044885 and NS42167 and the H. Houston Merritt Distinguished Professorship at the University of North Carolina School of Medicine.
NOTE: None of the PET radiopharmaceuticals mentioned in this article is FDA-approved for use in patients with cerebrovascular disease.
a Department of Neurology, University of North Carolina School of Medicine, 170 Manning Drive-Room 2131, CB #7025, Chapel Hill, NC 27599-7025, USA
b Department of Neurology, Washington University School of Medicine, 660 South Euclid Avenue, Box 8111, St Louis, MO 63110, USA
c Department of Radiology, Washington University School of Medicine, 510 South Kingshighway Boulevard, St Louis, MO 63110, USA
* Corresponding author.
E-mail address: powersw@neurology.unc.edu

Healthy young adults have an average whole brain cerebral blood flow (CBF) of approximately 46 mL $100g^{-1}$ min^{-1}, cerebral metabolic rate of oxygen ($CMRO_2$) of 3.0 mL $100g^{-1}$ min^{-1} (134 μmol $100g^{-1}$ min^{-1}), and cerebral metabolic rate of glucose (CMRglc) of 25 μmol $100g^{-1}$ min^{-1}.[5–8] The $CMRO_2$/CMRglc molar ratio calculated from arterio-jugular venous differences is 5.4 rather than 6.0, as expected for complete oxidation because of the production of a small amount of lactate by glycolysis.[5,7,9] CBF in gray matter (80 mL $100g^{-1}$ min^{-1}) is approximately 4 times higher than in white matter (20 mL $100g^{-1}$ min^{-1}), but differences of this magnitude are not seen with PET due to partial volume effects.[10] Under normal physiologic conditions, regional CBF is closely matched to the resting regional metabolic rate of the tissue.[11,12] As with CBF, $CMRO_2$ and CMRglc are higher in gray than white matter. Because of this relationship between regional flow and metabolism, the fraction of available glucose and oxygen extracted by the brain from the blood is uniform throughout the brain (**Fig. 1**). The oxygen extraction fraction (OEF) is normally 30% to 40%, indicating that oxygen supply is 2 to 3 times greater than oxygen demand. The glucose extraction fraction (GEF) is normally about 10%.[12,13]

Many studies report that CBF declines from the third decade onward.[14–17] The change in metabolic rate for oxygen and glucose with age is less clear, with several studies showing a decrease[14,16,18–20] and others showing no change.[21–23] Studies that have corrected for brain atrophy show lesser or absent changes in CBF, $CMRO_2$, and CMRglc with increasing age.[19,24–26] The authors' own PET data corrected for brain atrophy from 23 normal subjects, age 23 to 71 years, show no significant change in CBF or $CMRO_2$, but a decline in CMRglc of 4% to 5% per decade.

CEREBROVASCULAR CONTROL

Regional CBF is determined by the local cerebral perfusion pressure (CPP) and the local cerebrovascular resistance (CVR).

$$CBF = \frac{CPP}{CVR}$$

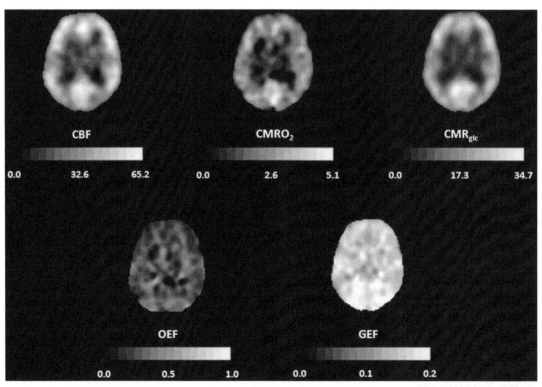

Fig. 1. Normal cerebral blood flow and metabolism. PET scans from a normal 70-year-old woman. Cerebral blood flow (CBF, mL $100g^{-1}$ min^{-1}), cerebral metabolic rate of oxygen ($CMRO_2$, mL $100g^{-1}$ min^{-1}), and cerebral metabolic rate of glucose (CMRglc; μmol $100g^{-1}$ min^{-1}) all show higher values in cortex that in white matter. Oxygen extraction fraction (OEF) and glucose extraction fraction (GEF) are relatively uniform throughout the brain. (*From* Powers WJ, Zazulia AR. The use of positron emission tomography in cerebrovascular disease. Neuroimaging Clin N Am 2003;13:742; with permission.)

CPP is equal to the difference between the mean arterial pressure (MAP) driving blood into the brain and the venous backpressure. Venous backpressure is negligible unless there is elevated intracranial pressure (ICP) or obstruction of venous outflow, such as cerebral venous thrombosis. Under normal conditions of constant MAP and CPP, any local changes in CBF must occur as a result of changes in CVR. CVR is determined by blood viscosity, vessel length, and vessel radius. Of these factors, changes in the radius of resistance vessels (primarily arterioles) are the primary determinants of CBF in most situations with normal CPP.

The cerebrovascular bed is not a static system. Resistance vessels dilate and constrict in response to a variety of stimuli. When there is a primary reduction in the metabolic rate of brain cells (eg, by hypothermia or barbiturates), vessels constrict to produce a comparable decline in CBF and thus little or no change in OEF or GEF.[27–29] With increased neuronal activity vessels dilate, producing an increase in regional CBF that is accompanied by a similar in magnitude increase in regional CMRglc and little or no increase in regional $CMRO_2$.[30–32] Acute changes in arterial pCO_2 cause proportional changes in CBF. A decrease in arterial pCO_2 from hyperventilation leads to a decrease in CBF (30%–35% at 25 mm Hg) and an increase in arterial pCO_2 leads to an increase in CBF (about 75% at 50 mm Hg).[33–37] The mechanism for the change in CBF is a change in CVR produced by vasodilation with increased pCO_2 and vasoconstriction with decreased pCO_2.[34] When the perturbation in arterial pCO_2 is maintained for a prolonged time, CBF gradually returns toward normal values.[37] With passive hyperventilation, no reduction in $CMRO_2$ or high energy phosphate levels accompanies the reduction in CBF.[38,39] However, with active hyperventilation, a slight increase in $CMRO_2$ has been reported.[33,34] The effects of arterial pO_2 on the cerebral circulation are different from those of pCO_2. CBF does not increase until arterial pO_2 is reduced to less than about 30 to 50 mm Hg,[40,41] indicating that variations in pO_2 are unlikely to constitute an important mechanism for regulating CBF at physiologic levels of pO_2. Because of the sigmoid shape of the oxygen dissociation curve, a significant reduction in hemoglobin saturation and hence in arterial oxygen content (CaO_2) does not occur until arterial pO_2 falls to about 50 to 60 mm Hg.[40,42] The similarity between this number and the threshold for hypoxia-induced reduction in CBF suggests that it is primarily CaO_2 and not pO_2 that determines CBF. Reductions in CaO_2 due to hypoxemia or anemia cause vasodilation and compensatory increases in CBF.[5,34,40,43] Likewise, the increase in CaO_2 with polycythemia is associated with a decrease in CBF.[44] In neither of these cases does cerebral metabolism change.[40,44] With chronic changes in CaO_2, there is a significant reciprocal inverse relationship between CaO_2 and CBF throughout the range of oxygen content levels such that oxygen delivery ($CBF \times CaO_2$) remains constant.[43] Acute changes in CaO_2 due to reduction in hemoglobin or pO_2 produce less of an increase in CBF than do chronic changes.[45,46] Hematocrit is an important determinant of viscosity and thus viscosity often varies with CaO_2. Although an inverse relationship between viscosity and CBF has also been reported,[43,47] it is unlikely that viscosity is an independent determinant of CBF under most circumstances. In anemic, paraproteinemic subjects in whom reduced CaO_2 is dissociated from changes in viscosity, there is no correlation between viscosity and CBF, but there is a highly significant inverse relationship between CaO_2 and CBF.[48] In hematologically normal subjects, reduction of viscosity by plasma exchange without a concomitant change in hemoglobin concentration or CaO_2 does not increase CBF.[49] Finally, reducing CaO_2 via carbon monoxide inhalation without changing arterial pO_2 or viscosity has been shown to increase CBF.[50] From these findings, it can be concluded that increases in blood viscosity induce compensatory vasodilation to maintain cerebral oxygen delivery. Thus, increases in CBF brought about by hemodilution, if they are simply reciprocal responses to changes in arterial oxygen content, will not increase cerebral oxygen delivery and may even decrease it.[51] This compensatory mechanism may be exhausted when preexisting vasodilation impairs the ability of vessels to dilate further to changes in viscosity.[52] All of these responses of the cerebral vasculature have been determined at normal CPP. When CPP varies, a different set of cerebrovascular and brain metabolic responses occur.

Changes in CPP over a wide range from 70 to 150 mm Hg have little effect on CBF. Known as autoregulation, this compensatory mechanism is mediated by changes in CVR. When CPP decreases, vasodilation of the small arteries or arterioles reduces CVR. When CPP increases, vasoconstriction of the small arteries or arterioles increases CVR.[53,54] This mechanism is effective at maintaining CBF in normal human subjects until MAP falls below the lower autoregulatory limit.[55,56] Chronic hypertension shifts both the lower and upper limits of autoregulation to higher levels. In chronically hypertensive subjects, the lower autoregulatory limit is 100 to 120 mm Hg MAP.[55,57] This limit is variably and unpredictably affected by chronic antihypertensive drug treatment. Thus, acute reductions in MAP or CPP that would be safe in normotensive subjects may precipitate cerebral ischemia in patients with chronic hypertension. As CPP falls below the autoregulatory limit and the maximal vasodilatory capacity of the cerebral circulation has been exceeded, there is a steep decline in CBF. A progressive increase in the amount of oxygen extracted from the blood by the brain by a factor of 2 or more to levels sometimes approaching 100% now maintains oxygen metabolism (**Fig. 2**).[58,59] When maximally increased OEF is no longer adequate to supply the energy needs of the brain, further reductions in CBF disrupt normal cellular metabolism and produce clinical evidence of brain dysfunction.

When the cerebral blood vessels are already dilated in response to some other stimulus, they are less responsive to further vasodilation induced by reduced CPP. Therefore, the autoregulatory response is attenuated or lost in the setting of preexisting hypercapnia, anemia, or severe hypoxemia.[60,61]

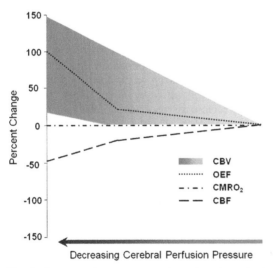

Fig. 2. Compensatory responses to reduced cerebral perfusion pressure (CPP). As CPP falls, cerebral blood flow (CBF) is initially maintained at almost baseline levels by arteriolar dilation. When vasodilatory capacity has been exceeded, cerebral autoregulation fails and CBF begins to decrease rapidly. A progressive increase in oxygen extraction fraction (OEF) preserves (CMRO$_2$). The response of cerebral blood volume (CBV) to reduced CPP is variable, ranging from a steady increase (of as much as 150%) to only a modest increase beginning at the point of autoregulatory failure. (*From* Powers WJ, Zazulia AR. The use of positron emission tomography in cerebrovascular disease. Neuroimaging Clin N Am 2003;13:743; with permission.)

The cerebral blood volume (CBV) is the amount of blood circulating in the brain vessels at any time. CBV is composed of arterial, capillary, and venous segments. Veins account for some 80% to 85% of CBV, arteries 10% to 15%, and capillaries less than 5%.[62,63] Of these, arteries are the most responsive to autoregulatory changes in CPP. Veins respond less and capillaries even less.[64,65] Although reductions in CPP produce visible dilation of pial vessels, data regarding the response of CBV to reduced CPP are conflicting[53,66–68] (see **Fig. 2**). With experimental reductions in CPP, it is sometimes possible to measure an increase in CBV that is presumed to be due to autoregulatory vasodilation.[69–71] However, this increase in CBV to reduced CPP is not always evident.[59] Failure to demonstrate increased CBV in the setting of reduced CPP has been ascribed to various possible mechanisms in various situations, including differential vasodilatory capacity of different vascular beds, passive collapse of vessels due to low intraluminal pressures, small vessel vasospasm, and resetting of vascular tone in response to a compensatory down-regulation of CMRO$_2$.[72] The CBF/CBV ratio (or its reciprocal, the mean vascular transit time, MVTT) has been proposed to be a more sensitive indicator of reduced CPP than CBV alone.[59,73] Although it may be more sensitive, it is not reliable because it may decrease in low flow conditions with normal perfusion pressure, such as hypocapnia.[74,75]

HEMODYNAMIC EFFECTS OF ARTERIAL OCCLUSIVE DISEASE

Carotid endarterectomy is empirically proven by randomized clinical trials to reduce subsequent stroke risk in patients with high-grade extracranial carotid stenosis; therefore, differentiating the relative importance of hemodynamic versus embolic mechanisms in these patients has little clinical value.[76,77] The same cannot be said for symptomatic carotid occlusion, for which no surgical treatment has proven to be effective in reducing the 5% to 10% annual risk of subsequent ipsilateral ischemic stroke on medical therapy.[2,78–80] A substantial amount of PET research has been devoted to assessing the hemodynamic effect of arterial occlusive disease with the goal of defining a subgroup of patients with hemodynamic compromise who might benefit from revascularization procedures.

The hemodynamic effect of carotid artery occlusion on the cerebral circulation depends on the adequacy of the collateral circulation. Vascular imaging techniques such as angiography or

Doppler ultrasonography can identify the presence of these collateral vessels, but not necessarily the adequacy of the blood supply they provide.[81]

Measurement of CBF alone also is inadequate for this purpose. First, normal CBF may be found when CPP is reduced but flow is maintained by autoregulatory vasodilation of distal resistance vessels. Second, CBF may be low when perfusion pressure is normal, such as when the metabolic demands of the tissue are reduced due to preexisting ischemic damage or the destruction of normal afferent or efferent fibers by a remote lesion.[58,82–84] Current methods for assessment of local cerebral hemodynamics depend on the compensatory responses observed during global reductions in CPP due to systemic hypotension and increased ICP, as described earlier. Similar responses are assumed to occur with local reductions in CPP due to focal arterial stenosis.

Three strategies are commonly used with PET to determine the hemodynamic effect of carotid artery occlusion on the cerebral circulation. The first relies on measurement of CBF at baseline and after application of a vasodilatory stimulus, such as CO_2 inhalation, acetazolamide administration, or physiologic increase in neuronal activity (eg, hand movement). Impairment of the normal increase in regional CBF to vasodilatory stimuli is assumed to reflect existing autoregulatory vasodilation due to reduced CPP. The second strategy entails the quantitative measurement of regional CBV either alone or in combination with measurement of CBF at rest to detect the presence of autoregulatory vasodilation. Increases in CBV or the CBV/CBF ratio relative to the range observed in normal control subjects are assumed to indicate hemodynamic compromise but, as noted earlier, the changes in CBV that can be measured with experimental reductions in CPP are variable and inconsistent. As a result, the sensitivity and specificity of these measurements in detecting reduced CPP is unknown. The third strategy involves direct measurement of regional OEF as an indicator of local autoregulatory failure.

Based on the known physiologic responses of CBF, CBV, and OEF to reductions in global CPP, a 3-stage sequential classification system for local cerebral hemodynamic status due to chronic carotid occlusion has been proposed.[85] Stage 0 is the condition of normal CPP due to collateral circulation that completely compensates for the occluded artery. CBF and $CMRO_2$ are closely matched such that OEF is normal. CBV is not elevated and the CBF response to vasodilatory stimuli is normal. Stage I hemodynamic compromise reflects a condition of reduced CPP whereby

CBF is maintained by autoregulatory vasodilation of arterioles. CBV consequently is increased and the CBF response to vasodilatory stimuli is decreased, but OEF remains normal. In Stage II hemodynamic failure, CPP is reduced to below the lower limit of autoregulation. There is increased OEF because CBF has declined with respect to $CMRO_2$. $CMRO_2$ is preserved at a level that reflects the underlying energy demands of the tissue, but may be lower than normal due to the effects of previous ischemic damage.[58,82,83] This stage has also been termed "misery perfusion" by Baron and colleagues (Fig. 3).[86,87]

Two independent PET studies have demonstrated that Stage II hemodynamic failure is a powerful independent predictor of subsequent ipsilateral ischemic stroke. Yamauchi and colleagues[88] found a significantly higher 1-year incidence of ipsilateral stroke in patients with symptomatic internal carotid artery (ICA) or middle cerebral artery (MCA) occlusive disease having increased OEF (4/7) than in those having normal OEF (2/33). In 3 of 4 patients with increased OEF and subsequent stroke, infarction occurred in a watershed territory corresponding to the area of increased OEF.[89] In the St Louis Carotid Occlusion Study (STLCOS), a blinded prospective study of 81 patients with symptomatic carotid occlusion, Grubb and colleagues[90] similarly found that increased OEF distal to the occlusion was an independent predictor of subsequent ipsilateral ischemic stroke. Ipsilateral stroke occurred in 11 of 39 patients with increased OEF and in 2 of 42 patients with normal OEF, respectively. When other factors were controlled for, patients with symptomatic carotid artery occlusion with increased OEF had a risk of ipsilateral ischemic stroke 7 times greater than those with normal OEF. These investigations establish the prognostic value of OEF in patients with symptomatic carotid occlusion but not its role in choosing therapy. Even though previous PET studies demonstrated improvement in OEF following extracranial-intracanial (EC-IC) bypass, the benefit of this surgery in reducing the risk of stroke remains to be determined by a properly designed clinical trial (see Fig. 3).[91–93] The Carotid Occlusion Surgery Study is currently underway to assess the efficacy of EC-IC bypass in reducing the risk of subsequent stroke in patients with symptomatic carotid occlusion who have increased OEF measured by PET.[94]

A PET study of patients with never-symptomatic carotid occlusion reported a lower incidence of elevated OEF (4 of 30) than is seen in symptomatic patients (39 of 81). Because no ipsilateral strokes occurred in any of the 30 subjects, no conclusions could be drawn with regard to the ability of

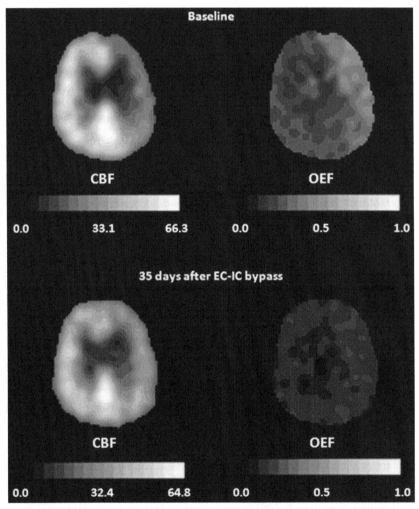

Fig. 3. Improvement of oxygen extraction fraction (OEF) after extracranial-intracranial (EC-IC) bypass surgery in a 69-year-old man with symptomatic occlusion of the right carotid artery. The baseline PET images (*top row*) demonstrate reduced cerebral blood flow (CBF, mL $100g^{-1}$ min^{-1}), and increased OEF in the right hemisphere. A second study performed 35 days after EC-IC bypass shows that ipsilateral CBF has improved and OEF has normalized (*bottom row*). In all images, the right side of the brain is on the reader's right. (*From* Powers WJ, Zazulia AR. The use of positron emission tomography in cerebrovascular disease. Neuroimaging Clin N Am 2003;13:746; with permission.)

increased OEF to predict ipsilateral stroke risk in this population.[95]

Although the 3-stage classification scheme is conceptually useful, it is too simplistic. As discussed earlier, increases in CBV are not reliable indices of reduced CPP. CBF responses to different vasodilatory agents may be impaired or normal in the same patient.[96–98] A normal vasodilatory response may occur in the setting of increased CBV.[99,100] Finally, according to the 3-stage system, all patients with increased OEF should have increased CBV and poor response to vasoactive stimuli. However, this increase in

CBV is not always evident nor is the impaired response to vasodilatory stimuli.[72,101]

In the original descriptions of the 3-stage classification of cerebral hemodynamics, the effects of further reductions in CPP and CBF when OEF is maximal (beyond Stage II) were described, but acknowledged to be based on inadequate data: $CMRO_2$ will decrease, normal cellular function and metabolism will be disrupted and cell death may occur. In this proposed scheme, OEF remained maximal as CBF and $CMRO_2$ both declined.[58,85] Nemoto and colleagues[102] have postulated that patients who initially have CPP below the autoregulatory limit with increased OEF (Stage II hemodynamic failure) may suffer subsequent ischemic neuronal damage that reduces $CMRO_2$ and normalizes OEF, but without any improvement in CPP. These investigators refer to this as Stage III. The plausibility of this scenario is supported by PET studies that show evidence for selective neuronal necrosis in brain regions with low $CMRO_2$ and normal OEF, and the progressive development of selective neuronal necrosis in areas with initially high OEF.[82,103] Nemoto and colleagues[102] propose that, while these patients would look like Stage I hemodynamic compromise (impaired response to vasodilatory stimuli, normal OEF), their stroke risk would in fact be similar to that of Stage II patients due to the persistently low CPP. Thus, according to this construct there should be a group of patients with normal OEF and impaired vasoreactivity who are at high risk for stroke. However, this does not seem to be the case. In the STLCOS, none of the 13 ipsilateral strokes that occurred in follow-up of 3.1 years occurred in patients with increased CBV and normal OEF.[72] The 2 patients with normal OEF who had ipsilateral strokes were among the 8 patients with the highest OEF values in the normal OEF group of 41 subjects. Furthermore, in this cohort of patients OEF was predictive of subsequent ipsilateral stroke as a continuous variable, indicating that the higher the OEF the higher the risk of stroke.[104]

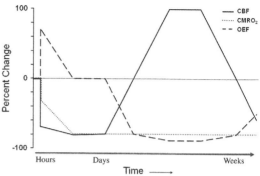

Fig. 4. Pathophysiological changes in cerebral infarction. At the onset of ischemia, the initial decrease in regional cerebral blood flow (CBF) is mirrored by an increase in regional oxygen extraction fraction (OEF). Because the increase in OEF is not sufficient to supply the energy needs of the brain, the regional cerebral metabolic rate of oxygen ($CMRO_2$) falls to the level of oxygen delivery. With time, $CMRO_2$ falls further even though there is only a slight further decrease in CBF, resulting in a decrease in OEF. Reperfusion via recanalization of the occluded artery or recruitment of collateral pathways results in an increase in CBF ("luxury perfusion") and a concomitant decrease in OEF to below baseline with no change in $CMRO_2$. With evolution to the stage of chronic infarction, CBF progressively declines and OEF increases, but often remains at less than baseline values. (*From Powers WJ, Zazulia AR. The use of positron emission tomography in cerebrovascular disease. Neuroimaging Clin N Am 2003;13:747; with permission.*)

EVOLUTION OF ACUTE INFARCTION

The evolution of changes in flow and metabolism early after acute ischemic stroke has been established from PET studies of MCA occlusion in large mammals. Approximately 1 hour after occlusion, CBF was decreased and OEF was increased in the territory of the occluded MCA. $CMRO_2$ was reduced somewhat initially in the deep regions of the territory, but fell further over the subsequent 2 to 3 hours. CBF remained relatively stable during this time period, falling only slightly.[105–109] Reflecting the stably reduced CBF and further declining $CMRO_2$, the initially markedly increased OEF progressively decreased. By 24 hours, CBF in the center of the MCA territory reached its nadir at less than 20% of baseline values and $CMRO_2$ reached 25% of baseline values (**Fig. 4**). Also at this time point, increased OEF was seen to develop outside the area of primary perfusion disturbance in the tissue adjacent to the infarct core.[109] The volume of severely hypometabolic tissue remained stable between 1 and 7 hours post occlusion, but increased by 24 hours and increased even further an average of 17 days after

occlusion.[110] The fate of high OEF regions in the core and surrounding regions is variable; some portions may go on to infarct and other portions may survive.[105]

Human data obtained at 2 to 24 hours after ictus show an area of reduced CBF, reduced $CMRO_2$, and high OEF.[111,112] Over the subsequent days, CBF usually increases. Spontaneous reperfusion will occur in about three-quarters of patients. Spontaneous reperfusion may take place within a few hours of infarction,[113] but peaks at day 14.[114] This increase in CBF occurs without a concomitant increase in $CMRO_2$; rather, $CMRO_2$ generally falls further. A consequent decrease in regional OEF below normal values mirrors the increase in CBF. This state, termed "luxury perfusion,"[115] indicates that the normal coupling of CBF to oxygen metabolism in the resting brain is deranged (**Fig. 5**). Luxury perfusion may be absolute with CBF values greater than normal. Alternatively, luxury perfusion may be relative, with low or normal CBF that is still in excess of that required to produce a normal OEF for the reduced $CMRO_2$.[116] Luxury perfusion is evident

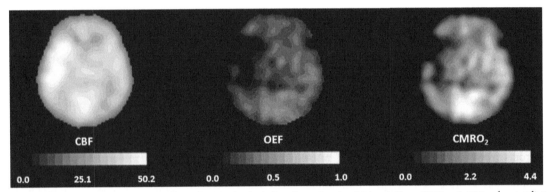

Fig. 5. Luxury perfusion 7 days after a hemispheric infarction. Cerebral blood flow (CBF, mL $100g^{-1}$ min^{-1}) is elevated in combination with reduced cerebral metabolic rate of oxygen ($CMRO_2$, mL $100g^{-1}$ min^{-1}) and OEF. (*From* Powers WJ, Zazulia AR. The use of positron emission tomography in cerebrovascular disease. Neuroimaging Clin N Am 2003;13:747; with permission.)

by 48 hours in one-third of patients[117,118] and peaks at 1 to 2 weeks, paralleling the time course of spontaneous reperfusion.[116] Following this subacute period, CBF progressively declines and OEF normalizes such that the chronic stable infarct demonstrates flow and metabolism that are close to zero with OEF at or below baseline values (**Fig. 6**).[119] In the rim of tissue surrounding the infarct core, areas demonstrating reduced CBF and increased OEF with variable $CMRO_2$ can often be identified within hours after ictus and may persist for up to 16 hours. As with the animal data, the fate of high OEF regions in the core and surrounding regions is variable; some will infarct and some will not.[120,121]

The peripheral benzodiazepine receptor ligand ^{11}C-PK 11195 primarily binds to cerebral microglia/macrophages.[122,123] This ligand can be used to image the inflammatory responses that occur following acute cerebral infarction.[124] In studies of human ischemic stroke, increased ^{11}C-PK 11195 uptake begins after 3 days and persists for months. Uptake is seen in the region of the primary lesion and later spreads to distant sites in the brain.[125,126]

IDENTIFICATION OF PREVENTABLE INFARCTION

Studies in experimental animals have elucidated the capacity of neurons to tolerate transient cerebral ischemia. At CBF less than 20 mL $100g^{-1}$ min^{-1}, neuronal electrical activity is at first impaired and then abolished. Neurologic deficits appear. If CBF remains below 20 mL $100g^{-1}$ min^{-1} the cells may go on to die. The ability of brain cells

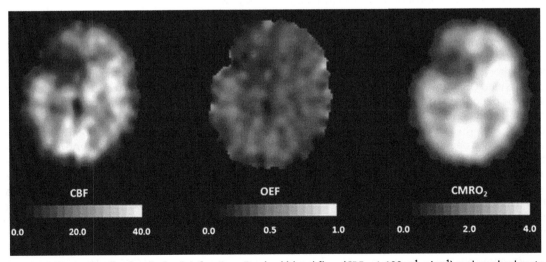

Fig. 6. PET 5 months after hemispheric infarction. Cerebral blood flow (CBF, mL $100g^{-1}$ min^{-1}) and cerebral metabolic rate of oxygen ($CMRO_2$, mL $100g^{-1}$ min^{-1}) are severely reduced, and oxygen extraction fraction (OEF) is below normal.

to tolerate CBF of less than 20 mL $100g^{-1}$ min^{-1} depends on both the magnitude and duration of the CBF reduction. CBF of 5 to 10 mL $100g^{-1}$ min^{-1} may be tolerated for a period of less than 1 hour, whereas CBF of 10 to 15 mL $100g^{-1}$ min^{-1} may not produce cell death for 2 to 3 hours. Some neurons may tolerate the same reduction in CBF for a period of time that is lethal to other cells. White matter is more tolerant than gray matter.[127–133] In a baboon model of transient MCA occlusion, evidence of reversibility as manifested by immediate improvement of hemiparesis was observed in 14 of 14 with occlusion less than 1 hour, 8 of 11 with occlusion of 2 to 4 hours, one-third with occlusion of 8 hours, and one-sixth with occlusion of 16 to 24 hours.[132,134–136]

The demonstration of improved recovery from stroke with early intravenous thrombolytic therapy provided the human counterpart for these experimental studies.[137,138] Although currently limited in practice to a time window of 4.5 hours, the variability observed in both animal experiments and clinical practice has led to a great deal of interest in developing a PET method to identify those patients with preventable infarction, that is, vulnerable brain cells that are still alive but whose natural history is to go on and die. A simple construct to test the ability of PET to accurately identify preventable infarction has recently been proposed (**Table 1**).[139] This construct requires 3 PET signals that spatially match the 3 pathophysiological tissue types in the brain with acute cerebral ischemia: already dead or irreversibly damaged (signal A), preventable infarction (signal B), and not at risk (signal C). Three distinct approaches based on 3 different PET radiopharmaceuticals have been investigated: ^{18}F-fluoromisonidazole (^{18}F-FMISO), ^{11}C-flumazenil (^{11}C-FMZ), and combined measurements of CBF and $CMRO_2$.

^{18}F-FMISO is a nitroimidazole compound that is selectively trapped within hypoxic but living cells.[140] Synthesis takes at least 1 hour and scanning cannot be performed until 2 hours after injection to provide adequate time for washout of unbound tracer.[140,141] Uptake of ^{18}F-FMISO PET was detected in the periphery and surrounding tissue of infarcts in 69% of patients studied within 48 hours and in no patient studied 6 to 11 days after stroke onset, including those who had positive early studies.[142] Uptake of ^{18}F-FMISO has been demonstrated to shift from the eventual infarct core (in patients studied <6 hours after stroke onset) to the periphery and surrounding tissue (in patients studied 6 to 48 hours after stroke onset). Over time, the amount of hypoxic tissue declines. When imaged within 6 hours of stroke onset, about 90% of the region of ^{18}F-FMISO is included in the eventual infarct whereas this percentage falls to 50% by 16 hours.[141,143] Clinical correlations exist between the volume of initially affected tissue and initial severity of the neurologic deficit and between the proportion of initially affected tissue progressing to infarction and neurologic deterioration during the first week after stroke.[143] During 2-hour transient MCA occlusion in the rat, the area of ^{18}F-FMISO uptake is much larger than the area of subsequent infarction, but a small area of infarction equal to 10% to 15% of the area of uptake still occurs.[144] Because a variable portion of the tissue detected by ^{18}F-FMISO uptake does not go on to infarct if untreated (more than 50% later than 16 hours after stroke onset), ^{18}F-FMISO does not accurately identify preventable infarction. The best interpretation for these data is that the degree of hypoxia necessary for ^{18}F-FMISO binding is less than the degree that leads to cell death.

^{11}C-FMZ is a central benzodiazepine receptor radioligand that binds to γ-aminobutyric acid (GABA) receptors on synapses of cortical neurons.[145] Because GABA receptors are sensitive to ischemia,[146] reduction of ^{11}C-FMZ uptake has been used to provide an early indication of neuronal damage.[146] A major limitation of the ^{11}C-FMZ technique is that the low or negligible densities of central benzodiazepine receptors in subcortical gray and white matter restrict its ability to detect tissue destruction in these regions.[147] Synthesis takes at least 1 hour and scanning takes 1 hour. In clinical ^{11}C-FMZ PET studies performed within 16 hours of stroke onset, decreased ^{11}C-FMZ binding was seen in areas of markedly decreased $CMRO_2$ despite a wide range of OEF values. ^{11}C-FMZ binding predicted final tissue status on late computed tomography (CT) with

Table 1
Criteria to establish accurate PET imaging of preventable infarction

	Imaging Signal A	Imaging Signal B	Imaging Signal C
Untreated tissue	All die	All die	All survive
Treated tissue	All die	All survive	All survive

a sensitivity of 84% and a specificity of 85%.[148] However, acute studies in the cat demonstrated that decreased ^{11}C-FMZ binding consistently underestimated the volume of subsequent tissue infarction.[149] In both tPA-treated and untreated patients, ^{11}C-FMZ binding of greater than 5.5 times contralateral white matter (CWM) is 95% predictive of late tissue survival, ^{11}C-FMZ binding of less than 3.4 times CWM is 95% predictive of late tissue death, and 3.4 to 5.5 times CWM is indeterminate. Combining with CBF measurements to improve the predictive value shows that ^{11}C-FMZ binding of more than 3.4 times CWM and CBF of less than 50% of contralateral hemisphere identifies tissue all of which will survive with thrombolysis for up to 3 hours, but that 80% will also survive if untreated.[2,148,150] Thus, ^{11}C-FMZ performs better than ^{18}F-FMISO, but still falls short at accurately identifying preventable infarction. Thresholds for 95% prediction of tissue death and survival can be derived as can accurate predictions of tissue survival with treatment. However, the fate of tissue with ^{11}C-FMZ binding between 3.4 and 5.5 times CWM is indeterminate. Most of the tissue with low CBF and high ^{11}C-FMZ binding that survives if treated will also survive when untreated.

Defining cells that are already dead or irreversibly damaged involves determination of thresholds for CBF or CMRO$_2$ below which spontaneous tissue survivability does not occur. Measurements of CBF alone perform poorly because of the importance of both magnitude and duration in determining cell death, the variable response of different cells, and the occurrence of high CBF in dead tissue (see earlier discussion).[121,151,152] Thresholds for cell death based on early measurement of CMRO$_2$ have been shown to be more reliable. CMRO$_2$ thresholds for infarction from 0.87 to 1.7 mL 100g^{-1} min^{-1} have been reported.[110,151,153,154] Identification of areas of preventable infarction by measurements of CBF and metabolism is much more difficult. Because tissue regions demonstrating increased OEF represent areas with reduced blood supply relative to oxygen demand but still with metabolically active cells, OEF has received much attention as the factor capable of predicting tissue viability, but it has been shown to be a poor predictor of tissue outcome.[105,121,152,155] The combination of CMRO$_2$ greater than 40% to 60% of normal and CBF les than 40% to 60% of normal has been shown to accurately identify areas of the brain that will go on to infarct if untreated and live if successfully reperfused. When both CBF and CMRO$_2$ are above these levels the tissue usually survives and when both are below these levels the tissue usually dies.[105–107,110,151,152,154–156] These data represent a mix from humans and nonhuman primates with minimal human reperfusion data. All these attempts to determine thresholds suffer from a variety of technical problems including small numbers of subjects, poor spatial resolution, lack of coregistration to CT, and poor counting statistics. Further human reperfusion studies are needed to demonstrate reliability of these criteria for identifying preventable infarction based on combined CBF and CMRO$_2$ in clinically heterogeneous patient populations.

CAROTID ARTERY ATHEROSCLEROSIS

Imaging of carotid atherosclerosis with ^{18}F-fluorodeoxyglucose (^{18}F-FDG) has demonstrated that plaques show varying levels of ^{18}F-FDG uptake.[157,158] The degree of uptake corresponds to pathologic evidence of active inflammation by macrophage infiltration.[159–161] The clinical relevance of these findings is still under investigation.[159,160,162]

REMOTE METABOLIC EFFECTS OF CEREBRAL INFARCTION

A common finding from PET studies of stroke is the presence of reduced blood flow and metabolism in brain regions distant from the site of infarction that appear normal on CT or magnetic resonance (MR) imaging. Remote hypometabolism has been demonstrated for both oxygen consumption[116,163–165] and glucose use.[166,167] Metabolic values at these distant sites always remain greater than those within the ischemic core.[112,166,167] CBF is reduced slightly more than metabolism, resulting in a slight increase in OEF.[168,169] Distinguished from "misery perfusion," this situation has been interpreted to represent primary metabolic depression with secondary reduction in perfusion.

The best-described remote metabolic effect of ischemia is contralateral cerebellar hypometabolism ("crossed cerebellar diaschisis"), which occurs in about 50% of patients with hemispheric lesions (**Fig. 7**).[165,170] Several factors have been reported to influence its occurrence, though data are not consistent across studies. Such hypometabolism may be more profound with greater volumes of hemispheric hypoperfusion,[171] deep MCA infarcts,[165] those involving the frontal[164] or parietal lobes,[116] and those encompassing more than one lobe.[165,167,172] Although Lenzi and colleagues[116] found that "crossed cerebellar diaschisis was not evident in cases in which the dimensions of the infarct were small," Martin and Raichle[164] reported no relationship to infarct size.

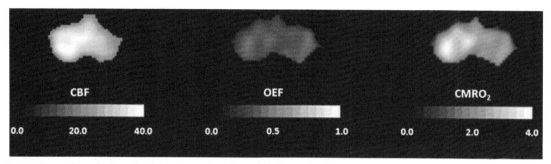

Fig. 7. Crossed cerebellar diaschisis 5 months after a left frontal infarct. Tomographic slices through the posterior fossa demonstrate reduced cerebral blood flow (CBF, mL 100g^{-1} min^{-1}) and cerebral metabolic rate of oxygen (CMRO$_2$, mL 100g^{-1} min^{-1}) in the right cerebellum. Oxygen extraction fraction (OEF) looks relatively uniform although it is usually found to be slightly elevated. In all images, the right side of the brain is on the reader's right.

Cerebellar hypometabolism has been shown to correlate with the presence of,[119] but likely not the severity of, hemiparesis.[164] This condition also occurs in some patients having no motor deficit.[165,167] Reduction of CMRglc is greater than that of CMRO$_2$ in chronic stroke (4 to 46 months), indicating an uncoupling of oxygen consumption and glucose use.[173]

Reduction in blood flow and metabolism in the hemisphere contralateral to cerebral infarction has also been described for both the homologous cortical area and for the whole hemisphere.[116,174,175] Wise and colleagues[176] found that although patients with recent infarction had lower contralateral CMRO$_2$ compared with normal control subjects, this difference vanished when the comparison group consisted of subjects with extracranial cerebrovascular disease but without previous cerebral infarction. Nonhuman primate models of cerebral ischemia have not revealed evidence for contralateral hemispheric hypometabolism either acutely[108] or at delayed measurement (>2 weeks).[155]

Ipsilateral cerebral hypometabolism has been observed in the cortex overlying subcortical stroke and in the basal ganglia, thalamus, and distant sites in the cortex after cortical stroke,[166,174,177,178] likely occurring in a delayed fashion (beyond 18 hours after clinical onset).[179] This "intrahemispheric remote hypometabolism" is most frequently described with thalamic lesions.[166,180,181]

These areas of remote hypometabolism are typically ascribed to a decrease in neuronal activity caused by interruption of afferent or efferent fiber pathways by the ischemic lesion, a phenomenon often termed *diaschisis*.[163] However, this term is not strictly accurate because diaschisis refers to an acute and reversible functional depression at sites distant from but connected with the site of injury,[182] whereas the remote effects of ischemia are often stable for months[164,183] and may be permanent. Trans-synaptic neuronal degeneration has been proposed as an alternate explanation for the remote hypometabolism[165] and is supported by the fact that contralateral CMRO$_2$ often declines between acute and chronic studies,[184] but this is unlikely to account for all cases, as hypometabolism can be seen within hours of stroke.[170,171] In the hemispheres distal to occluded carotid arteries, regions of reduced metabolism show evidence of reduced central benzodiazepine receptors consistent with selective neuronal damage.[82,185]

The clinical correlate of these remote changes is unclear. Single case reports have suggested an association with focal neurologic deficits, including ataxia,[186,187] aphasia,[188,189] neglect,[190] and hemianopia,[174] but larger series of infarcts at various locations have revealed no such relationships.[84,165] In one study, stepwise regression analysis revealed that language performance mainly depended on parieto-temporal metabolism irrespective of infarct location.[191] The relationship between remote metabolic effects seen acutely after stroke and eventual clinical outcome similarly is uncertain. Widespread metabolic disruption was a poor indicator of neurologic outcome (disability at 2 weeks to 3 months) regardless of CT findings in one study.[192] In another, metabolism in structurally normal ipsilateral mesial-prefrontal tissue at 5 to 18 hours after MCA stroke was predictive of neurologic status at 3 weeks.[179] Furthermore, glucose metabolism in the left hemisphere 2 to 3 weeks after left MCA stroke predicted both short-term (4 months) and long-term (2 year) recovery from aphasia.[193,194] The degree of acute crossed cerebellar hypometabolism did not correlate with the degree of later recovery in one study whereas in another it did.[170,171]

VASCULAR DEMENTIA

Vascular dementia remains an elusive entity. There are no agreed-upon clinical diagnostic criteria and the correspondence between the clinical diagnosis and pathology is poor.[195–197] The situation is further complicated by the common pathologic occurrence of both Alzheimer disease and cerebrovascular disease and their synergy in producing clinical dementia.[198] These cautions must be borne in mind in interpreting PET studies of vascular dementia, none of which have been based on pathologic diagnoses. These studies have primarily evaluated changes in CBF and $CMRO_2$ and, in some cases, used OEF to distinguish between ongoing active ischemia (high OEF) and permanent ischemic damage (normal or low OEF). Frackowiak and colleagues[199] reported reduced CBF and $CMRO_2$ and normal OEF in 9 subjects with vascular dementia, and concluded that there was no evidence to support the existence of a chronic ischemic brain syndrome. Similar findings were reported for patients with dementia associated with large cerebral infarcts.[200] Most of the other PET studies of vascular dementia have concentrated on patients with leukoaraiosis, the deep white matter abnormalities seen as hyperintensities on T2-weighted MR imaging and hypodensities on CT.[201,202] These abnormalities are associated with age-related cognitive decline.[202,203] Patients with leukoaraiosis have decreases CBF and $CMRO_2$ in both abnormal white matter and overlying gray matter, with the degree of reduction paralleling the severity of the white matter abnormalities and the degree of dementia. Both increased and normal OEF have been reported, leaving the issue of chronic ischemia unresolved.[200,204–207] Ihara and colleagues[207] have reported decreased cortical binding of ^{11}C-FMZ in patients with leukoaraiosis and dementia, suggesting that the white matter damage causes cortical neuronal injury.

INTRACEREBRAL HEMORRHAGE

Investigations of CBF and metabolic rate in intracerebral hemorrhage (ICH) have been less extensive than those in ischemic stroke. These studies have focused on the zone of tissue immediately surrounding the clot. Reduced CBF, determined by autoradiography or single-photon emission CT (SPECT), has been demonstrated in this area in experimental models of ICH[208,209] and in patients with ICH,[210] but not always.[211,212] This reduction in CBF is often attributed to cerebral ischemia due to mechanical compression of the microvasculature surrounding the clot.[208,213] As in ischemic stroke, PET and SPECT studies of ICH suffer from the effect of partial volume averaging, which may cause regions of normal flow to appear reduced depending on image resolution and the proximity to nonperfused tissue.[214,215] Unlike in ischemic stroke, a validated method exists permitting the correction for partial volume effects in ICH.[216] Using this method, a zone of hypoperfusion is still evident surrounding acute ICH.[216,217] In 19 patients studied 5 to 22 hours after symptom onset, Zazulia and colleagues[217] found that peri-clot $CMRO_2$ was reduced to a greater degree than CBF, resulting in decreased OEF rather than the increased OEF that occurs in ischemia (Fig. 8). This pattern was suggestive of a primary metabolic depression, consistent with a subsequent report of peri-hematomal mitochondrial dysfunction.[218] In 14 hypertensive patients with small- to medium-sized acute hemorrhages studied within 24 hours of onset, lowering MAP by 17% from 143 ± 10 to 119 ± 11 mm Hg did not produce any significant change in CBF in the peri-hematomal region or in the brain as a whole.[219]

Transient focal increases in glucose metabolism in the peri-hematomal region that occur 2 to 4 days after ICH have been described in 6 of 13 patients studied in the first week following ICH, who were resolving or had returned to baseline on repeat scans at 5 to 8 days (Fig. 9).[220] These focal increases are strikingly similar to foci of hyperglycolysis observed following traumatic brain injury.[221,222] Although the pathophysiological basis for these metabolic changes remains to be determined, they may indicate ongoing injury that is amenable to intervention that will improve outcome.[223] Remote hypometabolism in structurally intact brain regions, similar to that found with cerebral infarcts, is also seen in patients with ICH.[224,225]

ANEURYSMAL SUBARACHNOID HEMORRHAGE

Several PET studies performed within the first few days after aneurysm rupture have investigated the effects of subarachnoid hemorrhage (SAH) before vasospasm occurs. In one series of patients who had not undergone surgery and who did not have evidence for vasospasm, hydrocephalus, or ICH, there was a significant reduction in global $CMRO_2$ and CBF with normal OEF that did not correlate to the use of sedative drugs when they were studied 1 to 4 days after aneurysmal SAH.[226] This finding was interpreted by the investigators as indicating that the initial aneurysm

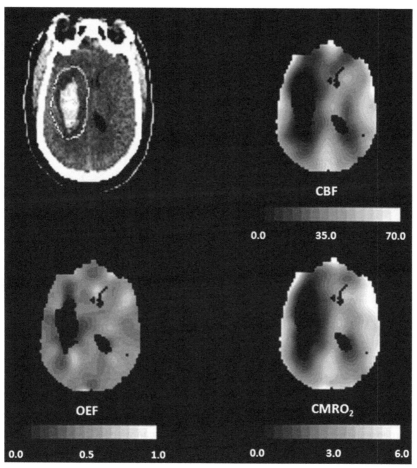

Fig. 8. PET images corrected for partial volume effects from a 44-year-old man with a putaminal hemorrhage studied 21 hours after onset. Peri-hematomal cerebral blood flow (CBF, mL $100g^{-1}$ min^{-1}), cerebral metabolic rate of oxygen ($CMRO_2$, mL $100g^{-1}$ min^{-1}), and oxygen extraction fraction (OEF) are all reduced compared with the contralateral hemisphere, indicating primary metabolic depression. (*From* Powers WJ, Zazulia AR. The use of positron emission tomography in cerebrovascular disease. Neuroimaging Clin N Am 2003;13:751; with permission.)

rupture produced a primary reduction in metabolism at this stage and the reduction in CBF occurred secondary to reduced metabolic demands. Another case series of 7 unsedated patients studied within the first 48 hours showed nonsignificant trends for a reduction in CBF and $CMRO_2$, and an increase in OEF. The investigators did not posit a causal relationship.[227]

Vasospasm, defined as segmental or diffuse narrowing of the large arteries at the base of the brain, can be detected angiographically in up to 70% of patients beginning at 4 to 12 days after aneurysm rupture.[228–230] Depression of CBF and $CMRO_2$ has been reported by several investigators with OEF variably described as normal or elevated.[231–237] Reduced metabolism with normal OEF has been interpreted as evidence for nonischemic primary metabolic depression with

vasospasm as a secondary response to reduced metabolic demand. However, because OEF returns to normal within several hours or at most a few days after cerebral infarction, the findings of normal OEF with reduced CBF and $CMRO_2$ cannot be used to discard ischemic infarction as a cause for reduced metabolism in SAH-induced vasospasm. Consistent with subacute cerebral infarction in which OEF had returned to normal, some investigators who have demonstrated reduced CBF and $CMRO_2$ with no change in OEF report subsequent cerebral infarction or moderate to severe disability in the majority of the patients.[234,235] To investigate whether large artery vasospasm causes ischemia without the confounding effects of subacute infarction, Carpenter and colleagues[226] studied a group of patients with vasospasm who did not develop subsequent

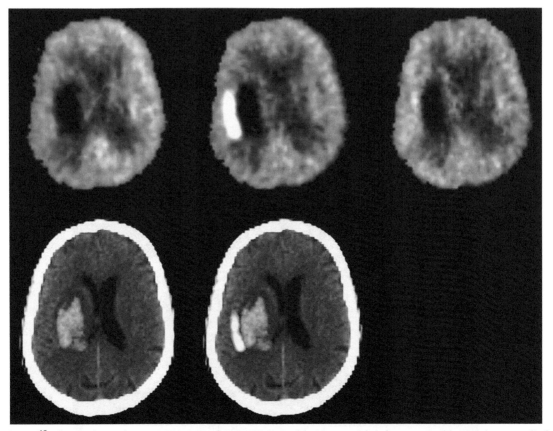

Fig. 9. ^{18}F-fluorordeoxyglucose PET images from a 72-year-old woman with left putaminal hemorrhage studied 26 hours (*top left*), 2.2 days (*top center*), and 4.9 days (*top right*) after onset. Images are normalized to mean activity in the initial scan. Bottom row shows initial CT (*left*) and the subtraction image of the first 2 PET studies superimposed on the CT, demonstrating the region of increased glucose metabolism adjacent to the hematoma.

infarction. CBF was decreased, $CMRO_2$ was normal, and OEF was increased, consistent with ischemia (**Fig. 10**).[226] With resolution of vasospasm, CBF increased.[236]

Studies of CBV in patients with SAH likewise have yielded conflicting results. In a non-PET study using oxygen-15 radiotracers, Grubb and colleagues[233] reported a statistically significant increase in CBV in patients of Hunt and Hess grade III to IV with angiographic vasospasm when compared with normal volunteers. OEF values were not reported, but examination of the CBF and $CMRO_2$ data indicates that OEF was probably not increased in the patients with vasospasm compared with those without. In a PET study of SAH, Hino and colleagues[234] reported a significant increase in CBV in regions of symptomatic angiographic vasospasm. These investigators did not, however, observe an elevation in regional OEF. In another PET study, patients with carotid artery occlusion were compared with those with SAH.[238] Regional OEF was higher, both during vasospasm and distal to carotid occlusion, than in SAH without vasospasm or in normal volunteers. Regional CBV was reduced compared with normal in regions with and without spasm, whereas it was increased ipsilateral to carotid occlusion. These findings of reduced CBV during vasospasm under similar conditions of tissue ischemia (increased OEF) that produce increased CBV in patients with carotid occlusion were interpreted as evidence that parenchymal vessels distal to arteries with angiographic spasm following SAH do not demonstrate normal autoregulatory vasodilation. The reason for the discrepancies among these studies in the measurement of CBV during vasospasm is not clear, but it may reflect the variability of CBV changes during reduced CPP noted earlier.[72]

Surgical retraction may have profound effects on cerebral metabolism. A small PET study before and after right frontotemporal craniotomies for clipping of ruptured anterior circulation aneurysms showed a 45% reduction in regional $CMRO_2$ and

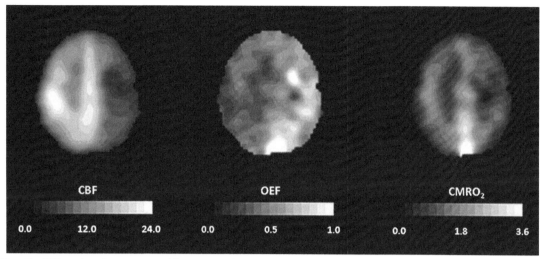

Fig. 10. PET study of a 54-year old woman who developed left hemiparesis due to vasospasm 9 days after subarachnoid hemorrhage. Right hemispheric cerebral blood flow (CBF, mL 100g^{-1} min^{-1}) is reduced more than the cerebral metabolic rate of oxygen (CMRO$_2$, mL 100g^{-1} min^{-1}) and oxygen extraction fraction (OEF) is increased, indicating ischemia. In all images, the right side of the brain is on the reader's right. (*From* Powers WJ, Zazulia AR. The use of positron emission tomography in cerebrovascular disease. Neuroimaging Clin N Am 2003;13:752; with permission.)

32% reduction in regional OEF without significant change in CBF in the region of retraction, but no change in the opposite hemisphere.[239] These changes indicate a primary reduction in metabolism and uncoupling of flow and metabolism (luxury perfusion). Such changes are not suggestive of vasospasm, because vasospasm produces diffuse changes respecting large vascular territories whereas these changes were focal in the area of retractor blade placement. Another study showed similar reductions in CMRglc in the area of retraction.[240]

SUMMARY

Measurements of CBF and CMR in ischemia and infarction have provided valuable insight into the pathophysiology of cerebrovascular disease. Much has been learned about the compensatory responses of the brain to reductions in perfusion pressure and in the evolution of changes in blood flow and metabolism that occur when these mechanisms fail. Knowledge of these changes can help guide therapy when multiple factors such as ischemia, hypoxemia, hypocarbia, or hypotension may be affecting CBF. Understanding the hemodynamic effects of arterial stenosis or occlusion on the downstream perfusion pressure has been instrumental in designing new trials for treatment.[94] In acute ischemic stroke, measurements of CBF and metabolism have been used to define the "ischemic penumbra" and to predict both

tissue and clinical outcome, although the clinical utility of these markers of ischemia in distinguishing viable from irreversibly damaged tissue in the acute period still requires further study.

Blood flow and metabolic studies in ICH have documented the integrity of autoregulation, and have suggested that hematomas exert a primary depression of metabolism rather than inducing ischemia in the surrounding tissue. This finding has important implications for future consideration of therapeutic interventions in this disease. Studies in SAH have differentiated the primary effects of the hemorrhage on cerebral hemodynamics and metabolism from those of vasospasm and surgical retraction. In addition, vasospasm-induced ischemia has been demonstrated to be reversible.

In summary, defining the pathophysiological changes in CBF and metabolism in human cerebrovascular disease has provided and will continue to provide the basic foundation for development and testing of new treatment strategies.

REFERENCES

1. Derdeyn CP, Videen TO, Simmons NR, et al. Count-based PET method for predicting ischemic stroke in patients with symptomatic carotid arterial occlusion. Radiology 1999;212(2):499–506.
2. Heiss WD, Kracht L, Grond M, et al. Early [(11)C]Flumazenil/H(2)O positron emission tomography predicts irreversible ischemic cortical

damage in stroke patients receiving acute thrombolytic therapy. Stroke 2000;31(2):366–9.

3. Siesjo BK. Brain energy metabolism. New York: John Wiley and Sons; 1978.

4. Rossen R, Kabat H, Anderson JP. Acute arrest of cerebral circulation in man. Arch Neurol Psychiatry 1943;50:510–28.

5. Cohen PJ, Alexander SC, Smith TC, et al. Effects of hypoxia and normocarbia on cerebral blood flow and metabolism in conscious man. J Appl Phys 1967;23(2):183–9.

6. Madsen PL, Holm S, Herning M, et al. Average blood flow and oxygen uptake in the human brain during resting wakefulness: a critical appraisal of the Kety-Schmidt technique. J Cereb Blood Flow Metab 1993;13:646–55.

7. Gottstein U, Bernsmeier A, Sedlmeyer I. Der Kohlenhydratstoffwechsel des menschlichen Gehirns bei Schlafmittelvergiftung. Klin Wschr 1963;41:943–8.

8. Scheinberg P, Stead EA. The cerebral blood flow in male subjects as measured by the nitrous oxide technique: normal values for blood flow, oxygen utilization, glucose utilization and peripheral resistance, with observations on the effect of tilting and anxiety. J Clin Invest 1949;28:1163–71.

9. Glenn TC, Kelly DF, Boscardin WJ, et al. Energy dysfunction as a predictor of outcome after moderate or severe head injury: indices of oxygen, glucose, and lactate metabolism. J Cereb Blood Flow Metab 2003;23(10):1239–50.

10. McHenry LC Jr, Merory J, Bass E, et al. Xenon-133 inhalation method for regional cerebral blood flow measurements: normal values and test-retest results. Stroke 1978;9(4):396–9.

11. Sette G, Baron JC, Mazoyer B, et al. Local brain haemodynamics and oxygen metabolism in cerebrovascular disease. Positron emission tomography. Brain 1989;112(Pt 4):931–51.

12. Baron JC, Rougemont D, Soussaline F, et al. Local interrelationships of cerebral oxygen consumption and glucose utilization in normal subjects and in ischemic stroke patients: a positron tomography study. J Cereb Blood Flow Metab 1984;4(2):140–9.

13. Lebrun-Grandie P, Baron JC, Soussaline F, et al. Coupling between regional blood flow and oxygen utilization in the normal human brain. A study with positron tomography and oxygen 15. Arch Neurol 1983;40(4):230–6.

14. Leenders KL, Perani D, Lammertsma AA, et al. Cerebral blood flow, blood volume and oxygen utilization. Normal values and effect of age. Brain 1990;113(Pt 1):27–47.

15. Kety SS. Human cerebral blood flow and oxygen consumption as related to aging. J Chronic Dis 1956;3:478–86.

16. Pantano P, Baron JC, Lebrun-Grandie P, et al. Regional cerebral blood flow and oxygen consumption in human aging. Stroke 1984;15(4):635–41.

17. Dastur DK. Cerebral blood flow and metabolism in normal human aging, pathological aging, and senile dementia. J Cereb Blood Flow Metab 1985;5(1):1–9.

18. Kuhl DE, Metter EJ, Riege WH, et al. The effect of normal aging on patterns of local cerebral glucose utilization. Ann Neurol 1984;15(Suppl):S133–7.

19. Marchal G, Rioux P, Petit-Taboue MC, et al. Regional cerebral oxygen consumption, blood flow, and blood volume in healthy human aging. Arch Neurol 1992;49(10):1013–20.

20. Yamaguchi T, Kanno I, Uemura K, et al. Reduction in regional cerebral metabolic rate of oxygen during human aging. Stroke 1986;17(6):1220–8.

21. de Leon MJ, George AE, Ferris SH, et al. Positron emission tomography and computed tomography assessments of the aging human brain. J Comput Assist Tomogr 1984;8(1):88–94.

22. Duara R, Margolin RA, Robertson-Tchabo EA, et al. Cerebral glucose utilization, as measured with positron emission tomography in 21 resting healthy men between the ages of 21 and 83 years. Brain 1983;106(Pt 3):761–75.

23. Duara R, Grady C, Haxby J, et al. Human brain glucose utilization and cognitive function in relation to age. Ann Neurol 1984;16(6):703–13.

24. Yoshii F, Barker WW, Chang JY, et al. Sensitivity of cerebral glucose metabolism to age, gender, brain volume, brain atrophy, and cerebrovascular risk factors. J Cereb Blood Flow Metab 1988;8(5):654–61.

25. Meltzer CC, Cantwell MN, Greer PJ, et al. Does cerebral blood flow decline in healthy aging? A PET study with partial-volume correction. J Nucl Med 2000;41(11):1842–8.

26. Ibanez V, Pietrini P, Furey ML, et al. Resting state brain glucose metabolism is not reduced in normotensive healthy men during aging, after correction for brain atrophy. Brain Res Bull 2004;63(2):147–54.

27. Astrup J, Sorensen PM, Sorensen HR. Oxygen and glucose consumption related to Na^+-K^+ transport in canine brain. Stroke 1981;12(6):726–30.

28. Bering EAJ, Taren JA, McMurrrey JD, et al. Studies on hypothermia in monkeys. II. The effect of hypothermia on the general physiology and cerebral metabolism of monkeys in the hypothermic state. Surg Gynecol Obstet 1956;102:134–8.

29. Nilsson L, Siesjo BK. The effect of phenobarbitone anaesthesia on blood flow and oxygen consumption in the rat brain. Acta Anaesthesiol Scand suppl 1975;57:18–24.

30. Sokoloff L. Relationships among local functional activity, energy metabolism, and blood flow in the

central nervous system. Fed Proc 1981;40(8): 2311–6.

31. Fox PT, Raichle ME. Focal physiological uncoupling of cerebral blood flow and oxidative metabolism during somatosensory stimulation in human subjects. Proc Natl Acad Sci U S A 1986;83(4): 1140–4.

32. Fox PT, Raichle ME, Mintun MA, et al. Nonoxidative glucose consumption during focal physiologic neural activity. Science 1988;241(4864):462–4.

33. Kety SS, Schmidt CF. The effects of active and passive hyperventilation on cerebral blood flow, cerebral oxygen consumption, cardiac output, and blood pressure of normal young men. J Clin Invest 1946;25:107–19.

34. Kety SS, Schmidt CF. The effects of altered arterial tensions of carbon dioxide and oxygen on cerebral blood flow and cerebral oxygen consumption of normal young men. J Clin Invest 1948;27:484–92.

35. Wollman H, Smith TC, Stephen GW, et al. Effects of extremes of respiratory and metabolic alkalosis on cerebral blood flow in man. J Appl Phys 1968; 24(1):60–5.

36. Fencl V, Vale JR, Broch JA. Respiration and cerebral blood flow in metabolic acidosis and alkalosis in humans. J Appl Phys 1969;27(1):67–76.

37. Raichle ME, Posner JB, Plum F. Cerebral blood flow during and after hyperventilation. Arch Neurol 1970;23(5):394–403.

38. Alexander SC, Smith TC, Strobel G, et al. Cerebral carbohydrate metabolism of man during respiratory and metabolic alkalosis. J Appl Phys 1968; 24(1):66–72.

39. van Rijen PC, Luyten PR, van der Sprenkel JW, et al. ^{1}H and ^{31}P NMR measurement of cerebral lactate, high-energy phosphate levels, and pH in humans during voluntary hyperventilation: associated EEG, capnographic, and Doppler findings. Magn Reson Med 1989;10(2):182–93.

40. Shimojyo S, Scheinberg P, Kogure K, et al. The effects of graded hypoxia upon transient cerebral blood flow and oxygen consumption. Neurology 1968;18(2):127–33.

41. Buck A, Schirlo C, Jasinksy V, et al. Changes of cerebral blood flow during short-term exposure to normobaric hypoxia. J Cereb Blood Flow Metab 1998;18(8):906–10.

42. Lassen NA. Cerebral blood flow and oxygen consumption in man. Physiol Rev 1959;39: 183–238.

43. Brown MM, Wade JP, Marshall J. Fundamental importance of arterial oxygen content in the regulation of cerebral blood flow in man. Brain 1985; 108(Pt 1):81–93.

44. Lambertsen CJ, Kough RH, Cooper DY, et al. Oxygen toxicity. Effects in man of oxygen inhalation at 1 and 3.5 atmospheres upon blood gas transport, cerebral circulation and cerebral metabolism. J Appl Phys 1953;5:471–86.

45. Todd MM, Wu B, Maktabi M, et al. Cerebral blood flow and oxygen delivery during hypoxemia and hemodilution: role of arterial oxygen content. Am J Phys 1994;267(5 Pt 2):H2025–31.

46. Mintun MA, Lundstrom BN, Snyder AZ, et al. Blood flow and oxygen delivery to human brain during functional activity: theoretical modeling and experimental data. Proc Natl Acad Sci U S A 2001; 98(12):6859–64.

47. Thomas DJ, Marshall J, Russell RW, et al. Effect of haematocrit on cerebral blood-flow in man. Lancet 1977;2(8045):941–3.

48. Brown MM, Marshall J. Regulation of cerebral blood flow in response to changes in blood viscosity. Lancet 1985;1(8429):604–9.

49. Brown MM, Marshall J. Effect of plasma exchange on blood viscosity and cerebral blood flow. Br Med J (Clin Res Ed) 1982;284(6331):1733–6.

50. Paulson OB, Parving HH, Olesen J, et al. Influence of carbon monoxide and of hemodilution on cerebral blood flow and blood gases in man. J Appl Phys 1973;35(1):111–6.

51. Hino A, Ueda S, Mizukawa N, et al. Effect of hemodilution on cerebral hemodynamics and oxygen metabolism. Stroke 1992;23(3):423–6.

52. Rebel A, Lenz C, Krieter H, et al. Oxygen delivery at high blood viscosity and decreased arterial oxygen content to brains of conscious rats. Am J Physiol Heart Circ Physiol 2001;280(6):H2591–7.

53. MacKenzie ET, Farrar JK, Fitch W, et al. Effects of hemorrhagic hypotension on the cerebral circulation. I. Cerebral blood flow and pial arteriolar caliber. Stroke 1979;10(6):711–8.

54. Symon L, Pasztor E, Dorsch NW, et al. Physiological responses of local areas of the cerebral circulation in experimental primates determined by the method of hydrogen clearance. Stroke 1973;4(4):632–42.

55. Strandgaard S. Autoregulation of cerebral blood flow in hypertensive patients. The modifying influence of prolonged antihypertensive treatment on the tolerance to acute, drug-induced hypotension. Circulation 1976;53(4):720–7.

56. Schmidt JF, Waldemar G, Vorstrup S, et al. Computerized analysis of cerebral blood flow autoregulation in humans: validation of a method for pharmacologic studies. J Cardiovasc Pharmacol 1990;15(6):983–8.

57. Strandgaard S, Olesen J, Skinhoj E, et al. Autoregulation of brain circulation in severe arterial hypertension. Br Med J 1973;1(852):507–10.

58. Powers WJ. Cerebral hemodynamics in ischemic cerebrovascular disease. Ann Neurol 1991;29(3): 231–40.

59. Schumann P, Touzani O, Young AR, et al. Evaluation of the ratio of cerebral blood flow to cerebral

blood volume as an index of local cerebral perfusion pressure. Brain 1998;121(Pt 7):1369–79.

60. Maruyama M, Shimoji K, Ichikawa T, et al. The effects of extreme hemodilutions on the autoregulation of cerebral blood flow, electroencephalogram and cerebral metabolic rate of oxygen in the dog. Stroke 1985;16(4):675–9.

61. Haggendal E, Johansson B. Effect of arterial carbon dioxide tension and oxygen saturation on cerebral blood flow autoregulation in dogs. Acta Physiol Scand 1965;66:27–53.

62. Wiedeman MP. Dimensions of blood vessels from distributing artery to collecting vein. Cirrulation Res 1963;12:375–8.

63. Hilal SK. Cerebral hemodynamics assessed by angiography. In: Newton TH, Potts DG, editors. Radiology of the skull and brain angiography, vol. 2, book 1. St. Louis (MO): C.V. Mosby Company; 1974. p. 1049–85.

64. Auer LM, Ishiyama N, Pucher R. Cerebrovascular response to intracranial hypertension. Acta Neurochir (Wien) 1987;84(3–4):124–8.

65. Kato Y, Auer LM. Cerebrovascular response to elevation of ventricular pressure. Acta Neurochir (Wien) 1989;98(3–4):184–8.

66. Fog M. Cerebral circulation. The reaction of pial arteries to a fall in blood pressure. Arch Neurol Psychiatry 1937;37:351–64.

67. Wolfe HG, Forbes HS. The cerebral circulation V. Observations of the pial circulation during changes in intracranial pressure. Arch Neurol Psychiatry 1928;20:1035–47.

68. Kato Y, Mokry M, Pucher R, et al. Cerebrovascular response to changes of cerebral venous pressure and cerebrospinal fluid pressure. Acta Neurochir (Wien) 1991;109(1–2):52–6.

69. Grubb RL Jr, Phelps ME, Raichle ME, et al. The effects of arterial blood pressure on the regional cerebral blood volume by X-ray fluorescence. Stroke 1973;4(3):390–9.

70. Grubb RL Jr, Raichle ME, Phelps ME, et al. Effects of increased intracranial pressure on cerebral blood volume, blood flow, and oxygen utilization in monkeys. J Neurosurg 1975;43(4): 385–98.

71. Ferrari M, Wilson DA, Hanley DF, et al. Effects of graded hypotension on cerebral blood flow, blood volume, and mean transit time in dogs. Am J Phys 1992;262(6 Pt 2):H1908–14.

72. Derdeyn CP, Videen TO, Yundt KD, et al. Variability of cerebral blood volume and oxygen extraction: stages of cerebral hemodynamic impairment revisited. Brain 2002;125:595–607.

73. Gibbs JM, Wise RJ, Leenders KL, et al. Evaluation of cerebral perfusion reserve in patients with carotid-artery occlusion. Lancet 1984;1(8372): 310–4.

74. Powers WJ. Is the ratio of cerebral blood volume to cerebral blood flow a reliable indicator of cerebral perfusion pressure? J Cereb Blood Flow Metab 1993;13(Suppl 1):S325.

75. Grubb RL Jr, Raichle ME, Eichling JO, et al. The effects of changes in $PaCO_2$ on cerebral blood volume, blood flow, and vascular mean transit time. Stroke 1974;5(5):630–9.

76. Executive Committee for the Asymptomatic Carotid Atherosclerosis Study. Endarterectomy for asymptomatic carotid artery stenosis. Executive committee for the asymptomatic carotid atherosclerosis study. JAMA 1995;273(18):1421–8.

77. Rothwell PM, Eliasziw M, Gutnikov SA, et al. Analysis of pooled data from the randomised controlled trials of endarterectomy for symptomatic carotid stenosis. Lancet 2003;361(9352):107–16.

78. Hankey GJ, Warlow CP. Prognosis of symptomatic carotid artery occlusion. Cerebrovasc Dis 1991;1: 245–56.

79. Klijn CJ, van Buren PA, Kappelle LJ, et al. Outcome in patients with symptomatic occlusion of the internal carotid artery. Eur J Vasc Endovasc Surg 2000;19(6):579–86.

80. Klijn CJM, Kappelle LJ, Tulleken CAF, et al. Symptomatic carotid artery occlusion: a reappraisal of hemodynamic factors. Stroke 1997;28:2084–93.

81. Derdeyn CP, Shaibani A, Moran CJ, et al. Lack of correlation between pattern of collateralization and misery perfusion in patients with carotid occlusion. Stroke 1999;30(5):1025–32.

82. Kuroda S, Shiga T, Ishikawa T, et al. Reduced blood flow and preserved vasoreactivity characterize oxygen hypometabolism due to incomplete infarction in occlusive carotid artery diseases. J Nucl Med 2004;45(6):943–9.

83. Kuroda S, Shiga T, Houkin K, et al. Cerebral oxygen metabolism and neuronal integrity in patients with impaired vasoreactivity attributable to occlusive carotid artery disease. Stroke 2006; 37(2):393–8.

84. Feeney DM, Baron JC. Diaschisis. Stroke 1986; 17(5):817–30.

85. Powers WJ, Press GA, Grubb RL Jr, et al. The effect of hemodynamically significant carotid artery disease on the hemodynamic status of the cerebral circulation. Ann Intern Med 1987;106(1): 27–34.

86. Baron JC, Bousser MG, Comar D, et al. Human hemispheric infarction studied by positron emission tomography and the ^{15}O continuous inhalation technique. In: Caille JM, Salamon G, editors. Computerized tomography. New York: Springer-Verlag; 1980. p. 231–7.

87. Baron JC, Bousser MG, Rey A, et al. Reversal of focal "misery-perfusion syndrome" by extra-intracranial arterial bypass in hemodynamic cerebral

ischemia. A case study with ^{15}O positron emission tomography. Stroke 1981;12(4):454–9.

88. Yamauchi H, Fukuyama H, Nagahama Y, et al. Evidence of misery perfusion and risk for recurrent stroke in major cerebral arterial occlusive diseases from PET. J Neurol Neurosurg Psychiatr 1996; 61(1):18–25.

89. Yamauchi H, Fukuyama H, Nagahama Y, et al. Significance of increased oxygen extraction fraction in five-year prognosis of major cerebral arterial occlusive diseases. J Nucl Med 1999;40(12):1992–8.

90. Grubb RL Jr, Derdeyn CP, Fritsch SM, et al. Importance of hemodynamic factors in the prognosis of symptomatic carotid occlusion. JAMA 1998; 280(12):1055–60.

91. Powers WJ, Martin WR, Herscovitch P, et al. Extracranial-intracranial bypass surgery: hemodynamic and metabolic effects. Neurology 1984;34(9):1168–74.

92. Gibbs JM, Wise RJ, Thomas DJ, et al. Cerebral haemodynamic changes after extracranial-intracranial bypass surgery. J Neurol Neurosurg Psychiatr 1987;50(2):140–50.

93. Samson Y, Baron JC, Bousser MG, et al. Effects of extra-intracranial arterial bypass on cerebral blood flow and oxygen metabolism in humans. Stroke 1985;16(4):609–16.

94. Adams HP Jr, Powers WJ, Grubb RL Jr, et al. Preview of a new trial of extracranial-to-intracranial arterial anastomosis: the carotid occlusion surgery study. Neurosurg Clin N Am 2001;12(3):613–24.

95. Powers WJ, Derdeyn CP, Fritsch SM, et al. Benign prognosis of never-symptomatic carotid occlusion. Neurology 2000;54(4):878–82.

96. Kazumata K, Tanaka N, Ishikawa T, et al. Dissociation of vasoreactivity to acetazolamide and hypercapnia. Comparative study in patients with chronic occlusive major cerebral artery disease. Stroke 1996;27(11):2052–8.

97. Inao S, Tadokoro M, Nishino M, et al. Neural activation of the brain with hemodynamic insufficiency. J Cereb Blood Flow Metab 1998;18(9):960–7.

98. Pindzola RR, Balzer JR, Nemoto EM, et al. Cerebrovascular reserve in patients with carotid occlusive disease assessed by stable xenon-enhanced ct cerebral blood flow and transcranial Doppler. Stroke 2001;32(8):1811–7.

99. Hirano T, Minematsu K, Hasegawa Y, et al. Acetazolamide reactivity on ^{123}I-IMP single photon emission computed tomography in patients with major cerebral artery occlusive disease: correlation with positron emission tomography parameters. J Cereb Blood Flow Metab 1994;14(5):763–70.

100. Nariai T, Suzuki R, Hirakawa K, et al. Vascular reserve in chronic cerebral ischemia measured by the acetazolamide challenge test: comparison with positron emission tomography. AJNR Am J Neuroradiol 1995;16(3):563–70.

101. Okazawa H, Tsuchida T, Kobayashi M, et al. Can the detection of misery perfusion in chronic cerebrovascular disease be based on reductions in baseline CBF and vasoreactivity? Eur J Nucl Med Mol Imaging 2007;34(1):121–9.

102. Nemoto EM, Yonas H, Kuwabara H, et al. Identification of hemodynamic compromise by cerebrovascular reserve and oxygen extraction fraction in occlusive vascular disease. J Cereb Blood Flow Metab 2004;24(10):1081–9.

103. Yamauchi H, Kudoh T, Kishibe Y, et al. Selective neuronal damage and chronic hemodynamic cerebral ischemia. Ann Neurol 2007; 61(5):454–65.

104. Derdeyn CP, Videen TO, Grubb RL Jr, et al. Comparison of PET oxygen extraction fraction methods for the prediction of stroke risk. J Nucl Med 2001;42(8):1195–7.

105. Giffard C, Young AR, Kerrouche N, et al. Outcome of acutely ischemic brain tissue in prolonged middle cerebral artery occlusion: a serial positron emission tomography investigation in the baboon. J Cereb Blood Flow Metab 2004;24(5):495–508.

106. Kuge Y, Yokota C, Tagaya M, et al. Serial changes in cerebral blood flow and flow-metabolism uncoupling in primates with acute thromboembolic stroke. J Cereb Blood Flow Metab 2001;21(3): 202–10.

107. Sakoh M, Ostergaard L, Rohl L, et al. Relationship between residual cerebral blood flow and oxygen metabolism as predictive of ischemic tissue viability: sequential multitracer positron emission tomography scanning of middle cerebral artery occlusion during the critical first 6 hours after stroke in pigs. J Neurosurg 2000; 93(4):647–57.

108. Pappata S, Fiorelli M, Rommel T, et al. PET study of changes in local brain hemodynamics and oxygen metabolism after unilateral middle cerebral artery occlusion in baboons. J Cereb Blood Flow Metab 1993;13(3):416–24.

109. Heiss WD, Graf R, Wienhard K, et al. Dynamic penumbra demonstrated by sequential multitracer PET after middle cerebral artery occlusion in cats. J Cereb Blood Flow Metab 1994;14(6):892–902.

110. Touzani O, Young AR, Derlon JM, et al. Sequential studies of severely hypometabolic tissue volumes after permanent middle cerebral artery occlusion. A positron emission tomographic investigation in anesthetized baboons. Stroke 1995;26(11):2112–9.

111. Ackerman RH, Lev MH, Mackay BC, et al. PET studies in acute stroke: Findings and relevance to therapy. J Cereb Blood Flow Metab 1989; 9(Suppl 1):S359.

112. Heiss WD, Huber M, Fink GR, et al. Progressive derangement of periinfarct viable tissue in

ischemic stroke. J Cereb Blood Flow Metab 1992; 12(2):193–203.

113. Molina CA, Montaner J, Abilleira S, et al. Timing of spontaneous recanalization and risk of hemorrhagic transformation in acute cardioembolic stroke. Stroke 2001;32(5):1079–84.

114. Jorgensen HS, Sperling B, Nakayama H, et al. Spontaneous reperfusion of cerebral infarcts in patients with acute stroke. Incidence, time course, and clinical outcome in the Copenhagen Stroke Study. Arch Neurol 1994;51(9):865–73.

115. Lassen NA. The luxury-perfusion syndrome and its possible relation to acute metabolic acidosis localised within the brain. Lancet 1966;2(7473): 1113–5.

116. Lenzi GL, Frackowiak RS, Jones T. Cerebral oxygen metabolism and blood flow in human cerebral ischemic infarction. J Cereb Blood Flow Metab 1982;2(3):321–35.

117. Hakim AM, Pokrupa RP, Villanueva J, et al. The effect of spontaneous reperfusion on metabolic function in early human cerebral infarcts. Ann Neurol 1987;21(3):279–89.

118. Marchal G, Serrati C, Rioux P, et al. PET imaging of cerebral perfusion and oxygen consumption in acute ischaemic stroke: relation to outcome. Lancet 1993;341(8850):925–7.

119. Baron JC, Bousser MG, Comar D, et al. Noninvasive tomographic study of cerebral blood flow and oxygen metabolism in vivo. Potentials, limitations, and clinical applications in cerebral ischemic disorders. Eur Neurol 1981;20(3):273–84.

120. Furlan M, Marchal G, Viader F, et al. Spontaneous neurological recovery after stroke and the fate of the ischemic penumbra. Ann Neurol 1996;40(2): 216–26.

121. Shimosegawa E, Hatazawa J, Ibaraki M, et al. Metabolic penumbra of acute brain infarction: a correlation with infarct growth. Ann Neurol 2005; 57(4):495–504.

122. Rojas S, Martin A, Arranz MJ, et al. Imaging brain inflammation with [^{11}C]PK11195 by PET and induction of the peripheral-type benzodiazepine receptor after transient focal ischemia in rats. J Cereb Blood Flow Metab 2007;27(12):1975–86.

123. Schroeter M, Dennin MA, Walberer M, et al. Neuroinflammation extends brain tissue at risk to vital peri-infarct tissue: a double tracer [^{11}C]PK1. J Cereb Blood Flow Metab 2009; 29(6):1216–25.

124. Myers R, Manjil LG, Cullen BM, et al. Macrophage and astrocyte populations in relation to [^{3}H]PK 11195 binding in rat cerebral cortex following a local ischaemic lesion. J Cereb Blood Flow Metab 1991;11(2):314–22.

125. Gerhard A, Schwarz J, Myers R, et al. Evolution of microglial activation in patients after ischemic stroke: a [^{11}C](R)-PK11195 PET study. Neuroimage 2005;24(2):591–5.

126. Price CJ, Wang D, Menon DK, et al. Intrinsic activated microglia map to the peri-infarct zone in the subacute phase of ischemic stroke. Stroke 2006; 37(7):1749–53.

127. Heiss WD, Rosner G. Functional recovery of cortical neurons as related to degree and duration of ischemia. Ann Neurol 1983;14(3): 294–301.

128. Marks MP, O'Donahue J, Fabricant JI, et al. Cerebral blood flow evaluation of arteriovenous malformations with stable xenon CT. AJNR Am J Neuroradiol 1988;9(6):1169–75.

129. Hossmann KA. Pathophysiology and therapy of experimental stroke. Cell Mol Neurobiol 2006; 26(7–8):1057–83.

130. Crockard HA, Gadian DG, Frackowiak RS, et al. Acute cerebral ischaemia: concurrent changes in cerebral blood flow, energy metabolites, pH, and lactate measured with hydrogen clearance and ^{31}P and ^{1}H nuclear magnetic resonance spectroscopy. II. Changes during ischaemia. J Cereb Blood Flow Metab 1987;7(4):394–402.

131. Astrup J, Symon L, Branston NM, et al. Cortical evoked potential and extracellular K$^+$ and H$^+$ at critical levels of brain ischemia. Stroke 1977;8(1): 51–7.

132. Marcoux FW, Morawetz RB, Crowell RM, et al. Differential regional vulnerability in transient focal cerebral ischemia. Stroke 1982;13(3):339–46.

133. Sundt TM Jr, Sharbrough FW, Piepgras DG, et al. Correlation of cerebral blood flow and electroencephalographic changes during carotid endarterectomy: with results of surgery and hemodynamics of cerebral ischemia. Mayo Clin Proc 1981;56(9):533–43.

134. Jones TH, Morawetz RB, Crowell RM, et al. Thresholds of focal cerebral ischemia in awake monkeys. J Neurosurg 1981;54(6):773–82.

135. Morawetz RB, Crowell RH, DeGirolami U, et al. Regional cerebral blood flow thresholds during cerebral ischemia. Fed Proc 1979;38(11):2493–4.

136. Crowell RM, Marcoux FW, DeGirolami U. Variability and reversibility of focal cerebral ischemia in unanesthetized monkeys. Neurology 1981;31(10): 1295–302.

137. Tissue plasminogen activator for acute ischemic stroke. The National Institute of Neurological Disorders and Stroke rt-PA Stroke Study Group. N Engl J Med 1995;333(24):1581–7.

138. Hacke W, Kaste M, Bluhmki E, et al. Thrombolysis with alteplase 3 to 4.5 hours after acute ischemic stroke. N Engl J Med 2008;359(13):1317–29.

139. Powers WJ. Imaging preventable infarction in patients with acute ischemic stroke. AJNR Am J Neuroradiol 2008;29:1823–5.

140. Nunn A, Linder K, Strauss HW. Nitroimidazoles and imaging hypoxia. Eur J Nucl Med 1995;22(3): 265–80.

141. Markus R, Reutens DC, Kazui S, et al. Topography and temporal evolution of hypoxic viable tissue identified by ^{18}F-fluoromisonidazole positron emission tomography in humans after ischemic stroke. Stroke 2003;34(11):2646–52.

142. Read SJ, Hirano T, Abbott DF, et al. Identifying hypoxic tissue after acute ischemic stroke using PET and ^{18}F-fluoromisonidazole. Neurology 1998; 51(6):1617–21.

143. Read SJ, Hirano T, Abbott DF, et al. The fate of hypoxic tissue on ^{18}F-fluoromisonidazole positron emission tomography after ischemic stroke. Ann Neurol 2000;48(2):228–35.

144. Saita K, Chen M, Spratt NJ, et al. Imaging the ischemic penumbra with ^{18}F-fluoromisonidazole in a rat model of ischemic stroke. Stroke 2004;35(4): 975–80.

145. Hantraye P, Kaijima M, Prenant C, et al. Central type benzodiazepine binding sites: a positron emission tomography study in the baboon's brain. Neurosci Lett 1984;48(2):115–20.

146. Schwartz RD, Yu X, Wagner J, et al. Cellular regulation of the benzodiazepine/GABA receptor: arachidonic acid, calcium, and cerebral ischemia. Neuropsychopharmacology 1992;6(2):119–25.

147. Abadie P, Baron JC, Bisserbe JC, et al. Central benzodiazepine receptors in human brain: estimation of regional B_{max} and K_D values with positron emission tomography. Eur J Pharmacol 1992; 213(1):107–15.

148. Heiss WD, Grond M, Thiel A, et al. Permanent cortical damage detected by flumazenil positron emission tomography in acute stroke. Stroke 1998;29(2):454–61.

149. Heiss WD, Graf R, Fujita T, et al. Early detection of irreversibly damaged ischemic tissue by flumazenil positron emission tomography in cats. Stroke 1997; 28(10):2045–51.

150. Heiss WD, Kracht LW, Thiel A, et al. Penumbral probability thresholds of cortical flumazenil binding and blood flow predicting tissue outcome in patients with cerebral ischemia. Brain 2001;124:20–9.

151. Powers WJ, Grubb RL Jr, Darriet D, et al. Cerebral blood flow and cerebral metabolic rate of oxygen requirements for cerebral function and viability in humans. J Cereb Blood Flow Metab 1985;5(4): 600–8.

152. Frykholm P, Andersson JL, Valtysson J, et al. A metabolic threshold of irreversible ischemia demonstrated by PET in a middle cerebral artery occlusion-reperfusion primate model. Acta Neurol Scand 2000;102(1):18–26.

153. Baron JC, Rougemont D, Bousser MG, et al. Oxygen extraction fraction (OEF), and $CMRO_2$: prognostic value in recent supratentorial infarction in humans. J Cereb Blood Flow Metab 1983; 3(Suppl 1):S1–2.

154. Marchal G, Benali K, Iglesias S, et al. Voxel-based mapping of irreversible ischaemic damage with PET in acute stroke. Brain 1999;122(Pt 12):2387–400.

155. Young AR, Sette G, Touzani O, et al. Relationships between high oxygen extraction fraction in the acute stage and final infarction in reversible middle cerebral artery occlusion: an investigation in anesthetized baboons with positron emission tomography. J Cereb Blood Flow Metab 1996;16(6):1176–88.

156. Marchal G, Beaudouin V, Rioux P, et al. Prolonged persistence of substantial volumes of potentially viable brain tissue after stroke: a correlative PET-CT study with voxel-based data analysis. Stroke 1996;27(4):599–606.

157. Yun M, Yeh D, Araujo LI, et al. F-18 FDG uptake in the large arteries: a new observation. Clin Nucl Med 2001;26(4):314–9.

158. Rudd JH, Warburton EA, Fryer TD, et al. Imaging atherosclerotic plaque inflammation with ^{18}F-fluorodeoxyglucose positron emission tomography. Circulation 2002;105(23):2708–11.

159. Tawakol A, Migrino RQ, Bashian GG, et al. In vivo ^{18}F-fluorodeoxyglucose positron emission tomography imaging provides a noninvasive measure of carotid plaque inflammation in patients. J Am Coll Cardiol 2006;48(9):1818–24.

160. Font MA, Fernandez A, Carvajal A, et al. Imaging of early inflammation in low-to-moderate carotid stenosis by 18-FDG-PET. Front Biosci 2009;14: 3352–60.

161. Graebe M, Pedersen SF, Borgwardt L, et al. Molecular pathology in vulnerable carotid plaques: correlation with [18]-fluorodeoxyglucose positron emission tomography (FDG-PET). Eur J Vasc Endovasc Surg 2009;37(6):714–21.

162. Davies JR, Rudd JH, Fryer TD, et al. Identification of culprit lesions after transient ischemic attack by combined ^{18}F fluorodeoxyglucose positron-emission tomography and high-resolution magnetic resonance imaging. Stroke 2005;36(12):2642–7.

163. Baron JC, Bousser MG, Comar D, et al. 'Crossed cerebellar diaschisis' in human supratentorial brain infarction. Trans Am Neurol Assoc 1980;105:459–61.

164. Martin WR, Raichle ME. Cerebellar blood flow and metabolism in cerebral hemisphere infarction. Ann Neurol 1983;14(2):168–76.

165. Pantano P, Baron JC, Samson Y, et al. Crossed cerebellar diaschisis. Further studies. Brain 1986; 109(Pt 4):677–94.

166. Kuhl DE, Phelps ME, Kowell AP, et al. Effects of stroke on local cerebral metabolism and perfusion: mapping by emission computed tomography of [18]FDG and [13]NH_3. Ann Neurol 1980;8(1):47–60.

167. Kushner M, Alavi A, Reivich M, et al. Contralateral cerebellar hypometabolism following cerebral insult: a positron emission tomographic study. Ann Neurol 1984;15(5):425–34.

168. Ito H, Kanno I, Shimosegawa E, et al. Hemodynamic changes during neural deactivation in human brain: a positron emission tomography study of crossed cerebellar diaschisis. Ann Nucl Med 2002;16(4):249–54.

169. Yamauchi H, Fukuyama H, Kimura J. Hemodynamic and metabolic changes in crossed cerebellar hypoperfusion. Stroke 1992;23(6):855–60.

170. Serrati C, Marchal G, Rioux P, et al. Contralateral cerebellar hypometabolism: a predictor for stroke outcome? J Neurol Neurosurg Psychiatr 1994; 57(2):174–9.

171. Sobesky J, Thiel A, Ghaemi M, et al. Crossed cerebellar diaschisis in acute human stroke: a PET study of serial changes and response to supratentorial reperfusion. J Cereb Blood Flow Metab 2005; 25(12):1685–91.

172. Kim SE, Choi CW, Yoon BW, et al. Crossed-cerebellar diaschisis in cerebral infarction: technetium-99m-HMPAO SPECT and MRI. J Nucl Med 1997;38(1):14–9.

173. Yamauchi H, Fukuyama H, Nagahama Y, et al. Uncoupling of oxygen and glucose metabolism in persistent crossed cerebellar diaschisis. Stroke 1999;30(7):1424–8.

174. Celesia GG, Polcyn RE, Holden JE, et al. Determination of regional cerebral blood flow in patients with cerebral infarction. Use of fluoromethane labeled with fluorine 18 and positron emission tomography. Arch Neurol 1984;41(3):262–7.

175. Dobkin JA, Levine RL, Lagreze HL, et al. Evidence for transhemispheric diaschisis in unilateral stroke. Arch Neurol 1989;46(12):1333–6.

176. Wise R, Gibbs J, Frackowiak R, et al. No evidence for transhemispheric diaschisis after human cerebral infarction. Stroke 1986;17(5):853–61.

177. Baron JC, Lebrun-Grandie P, Collard P, et al. Noninvasive measurement of blood flow, oxygen consumption, and glucose utilization in the same brain regions in man by positron emission tomography: concise communication. J Nucl Med 1982; 23(5):391–9.

178. Heiss WD, Pawlik G, Wagner R, et al. Functional hypometabolism of noninfarcted brain regions in ischemic stroke. J Cereb Blood Flow Metab 1983; 3(Suppl 1):S582–3.

179. Iglesias S, Marchal G, Viader F, et al. Delayed intrahemispheric remote hypometabolism. Correlations with early recovery after stroke. Cerebrovasc Dis 2000;10(5):391–402.

180. Wise RJ, Bernardi S, Frackowiak RS, et al. Serial observations on the pathophysiology of acute stroke. The transition from ischaemia to infarction as reflected in regional oxygen extraction. Brain 1983;106(Pt 1):197–222.

181. Szelies B, Herholz K, Pawlik G, et al. Widespread functional effects of discrete thalamic infarction. Arch Neurol 1991;48(2):178–82.

182. Von Monakow C. Diaschisis. In: Pribram KA, editor. Brain and behavior I: mood, states and mind. Baltimore (MD): Penguin Books; 1969. p. 27–36.

183. Lenzi GL, Frackowiak RS, Jones T, et al. $CMRO_2$ and CBF by the oxygen-15 inhalation technique. Results in normal volunteers and cerebrovascular patients. Eur Neurol 1981;20(3):285–90.

184. Iglesias S, Marchal G, Rioux P, et al. Do changes in oxygen metabolism in the unaffected cerebral hemisphere underlie early neurological recovery after stroke? A positron emission tomography study. Stroke 1996;27(7):1192–9.

185. Dong Y, Fukuyama H, Nabatame H, et al. Assessment of benzodiazepine receptors using iodine-123-labeled iomazenil single-photon emission computed tomography in patients with ischemic cerebrovascular disease. A comparison with PET study. Stroke 1997;28(9):1776–82.

186. Sakai F, Aoki S, Kan S, et al. Ataxic hemiparesis with reductions of ipsilateral cerebellar blood flow. Stroke 1986;17(5):1016–8.

187. Giroud M, Creisson E, Fayolle H, et al. Homolateral ataxia and crural paresis: a crossed cerebral-cerebellar diaschisis. J Neurol Neurosurg Psychiatr 1994;57(2):221–2.

188. Metter EJ, Kempler D, Jackson C, et al. Cerebral glucose metabolism in Wernicke's, Broca's, and conduction aphasia. Arch Neurol 1989;46(1):27–34.

189. Karbe H, Herholz K, Szelies B, et al. Regional metabolic correlates of Token test results in cortical and subcortical left hemispheric infarction. Neurology 1989;39(8):1083–8.

190. Perani D, Vallar G, Cappa S, et al. Aphasia and neglect after subcortical stroke. A clinical/cerebral perfusion correlation study. Brain 1987;110(Pt 5): 1211–29.

191. Karbe H, Szelies B, Herholz K, et al. Impairment of language is related to left parieto-temporal glucose metabolism in aphasic stroke patients. J Neurol 1990;237(1):19–23.

192. Kushner M, Reivich M, Fieschi C, et al. Metabolic and clinical correlates of acute ischemic infarction. Neurology 1987;37(7):1103–10.

193. Heiss WD, Kessler J, Karbe H, et al. Cerebral glucose metabolism as a predictor of recovery from aphasia in ischemic stroke. Arch Neurol 1993;50(9):958–64.

194. Karbe H, Kessler J, Herholz K, et al. Long-term prognosis of poststroke aphasia studied with positron emission tomography. Arch Neurol 1995;52(2): 186–90.

195. Chui HC, Mack W, Jackson JE, et al. Clinical criteria for the diagnosis of vascular dementia: a multicenter study of comparability and interrater reliability. Arch Neurol 2000;57(2):191–6.

196. Brunnstrom H, Englund E. Clinicopathological concordance in dementia diagnostics. Am J Geriatr Psychiatry 2009;17(8):664–70.

197. Lopez OL, Kuller LH, Becker JT, et al. Classification of vascular dementia in the Cardiovascular Health Study Cognition Study. Neurology 2005;64(9): 1539–47.

198. Smith CD, Snowdon DA, Wang H, et al. White matter volumes and periventricular white matter hyperintensities in aging and dementia. Neurology 2000;54(4):838–42.

199. Frackowiak RS, Pozzilli C, Legg NJ, et al. Regional cerebral oxygen supply and utilization in dementia. A clinical and physiological study with oxygen-15 and positron tomography. Brain 1981;104(Pt 4): 753–78.

200. De Reuck J, Decoo D, Marchau M, et al. Positron emission tomography in vascular dementia. J Neurol Sci 1998;154(1):55–61.

201. Hachinski VC, Potter P, Merskey H. Leuko-araiosis. Arch Neurol 1987;44(1):21–3.

202. Schmidt R, Petrovic K, Ropele S, et al. Progression of leukoaraiosis and cognition. Stroke 2007;38(9): 2619–25.

203. Pantoni L, Poggesi A, Inzitari D. The relation between white-matter lesions and cognition. Curr Opin Neurol 2007;20(4):390–7.

204. Tohgi H, Yonezawa H, Takahashi S, et al. Cerebral blood flow and oxygen metabolism in senile dementia of Alzheimer's type and vascular dementia with deep white matter changes. Neuroradiology 1998;40(3):131–7.

205. Meguro K, Hatazawa J, Yamaguchi T, et al. Cerebral circulation and oxygen metabolism associated with subclinical periventricular hyperintensity as shown by magnetic resonance imaging. Ann Neurol 1990;28(3):378–83.

206. De Reuck J, Decoo D, Strijckmans K, et al. Does the severity of leukoaraiosis contribute to senile dementia? A comparative computerized and positron emission tomographic study. Eur Neurol 1992;32(4):199–205.

207. Ihara M, Tomimoto H, Ishizu K, et al. Decrease in cortical benzodiazepine receptors in symptomatic patients with leukoaraiosis: a positron emission tomography study. Stroke 2004;35(4):942–7.

208. Mendelow AD, Bullock R, Teasdale GM, et al. Intracranial haemorrhage induced at arterial pressure in the rat. Part 2: short term changes in local cerebral blood flow measured by autoradiography. Neurol Res 1984;6(4):189–93.

209. Nath FP, Jenkins A, Mendelow AD, et al. Early hemodynamic changes in experimental intracerebral hemorrhage. J Neurosurg 1986; 65(5):697–703.

210. Sills C, Villar-Cordova C, Pasteur W, et al. Demonstration of hypoperfusion surrounding intracerebral hematoma in humans. J Stroke Cerebrovasc Dis 1996;6:17–24.

211. Qureshi AI, Wilson DA, Hanley DF, et al. No evidence for an ischemic penumbra in massive experimental intracerebral hemorrhage. Neurology 1999;52(2):266–72.

212. Mayer SA, Lignelli A, Fink MF, et al. Perilesional blood flow and edema formation in acute intracerebral hemorrhage: a SPECT study. Stroke 1998; 29(9):1791–8.

213. Nath FP, Kelly PT, Jenkins A, et al. Effects of experimental intracerebral hemorrhage on blood flow, capillary permeability, and histochemistry. J Neurosurg 1987;66(4):555–62.

214. Hoffman EJ, Huang SC, Phelps ME. Quantitation in positron emission computed tomography: 1. Effect of object size. J Comput Assist Tomogr 1979;3(3): 299–308.

215. Mazziotta JC, Phelps ME, Plummer D, et al. Quantitation in positron emission computed tomography: 5. Physical-anatomical effects. J Comput Assist Tomogr 1981;5(5):734–43.

216. Videen TO, Dunford-Shore JE, Diringer MN, et al. Correction for partial volume effects in regional blood flow measurements adjacent to hematomas in humans with intracerebral hemorrhage: implementation and validation. J Comput Assist Tomogr 1999;23(2):248–56.

217. Zazulia AR, Diringer MN, Videen TO, et al. Hypoperfusion without ischemia surrounding acute intracerebral hemorrhage. J Cereb Blood Flow Metab 2001;21:804–10.

218. Kim-Han JS, Kopp SJ, Dugan LL, et al. Perihematomal mitochondrial dysfunction after intracerebral hemorrhage. Stroke 2006;37(10):2457–62.

219. Powers WJ, Zazulia AR, Videen TO, et al. Autoregulation of cerebral blood flow surrounding acute (6 to 22 hours) intracerebral hemorrhage. Neurology 2001;57(1):18–24.

220. Zazulia AR, Videen TO, Powers WJ. Transient focal increase in perihematomal glucose metabolism after acute human intracerebral hemorrhage. Stroke 2009;40(5):1638–43.

221. Bergsneider M, Hovda DA, Shalmon E, et al. Cerebral hyperglycolysis following severe traumatic brain injury in humans: a positron emission tomography study. J Neurosurg 1997;86(2):241–51.

222. Hattori N, Huang SC, Wu HM, et al. Acute changes in regional cerebral (^{18})F-FDG kinetics in patients with traumatic brain injury. J Nucl Med 2004; 45(5):775–83.

223. Vespa PM. Metabolic penumbra in intracerebral hemorrhage. Stroke 2009;40(5):1547–8.

224. Heiss WD, Beil C, Pawlik G, et al. Non-traumatic intracerebral hematoma versus ischemic stroke: regional pattern of glucose metabolism. J Cereb Blood Flow Metab 1985;5(Suppl 1):S5–6.

225. Dal-Bianco P. Positron emission tomography of 2(^{18}F)-fluorodeoxyglucose in cerebral vascular disease: clinicometabolic correlations in patients with nontraumatic spontaneous intracerebral hematoma and ischemic infarction. In: Meyer JS, Lechner H, Reivich M, Ott EO, editors. Cerebral vascular disease 6: proceedings of the world federation of neurology 13th International Salzburg conference. Amsterdam: Excerpta Medica; 1987. p. 257–62.

226. Carpenter DA, Grubb RL Jr, Tempel LW, et al. Cerebral oxygen metabolism after aneurysmal subarachnoid hemorrhage. J Cereb Blood Flow Metab 1991;11(5):837–44.

227. Frykholm P, Andersson JL, Langstrom B, et al. Haemodynamic and metabolic disturbances in the acute stage of subarachnoid haemorrhage demonstrated by PET. Acta Neurol Scand 2004;109(1):25–32.

228. Kassell NF, Sasaki T, Colohan AR, et al. Cerebral vasospasm following aneurysmal subarachnoid hemorrhage. Stroke 1985;16(4):562–72.

229. Heros RC, Zervas NT, Varsos V. Cerebral vasospasm after subarachnoid hemorrhage: an update. Ann Neurol 1983;14(6):599–608.

230. Suarez JI, Tarr RW, Selman WR. Aneurysmal subarachnoid hemorrhage. N Engl J Med 2006; 354(4):387–96.

231. Jakobsen M, Enevoldsen E, Bjerre P. Cerebral blood flow and metabolism following subarachnoid haemorrhage: cerebral oxygen uptake and global blood flow during the acute period in patients with SAH. Acta Neurol Scand 1990;82(3):174–82.

232. Hayashi T, Suzuki A, Hatazawa J, et al. Cerebral circulation and metabolism in the acute stage of subarachnoid hemorrhage. J Neurosurg 2000; 93(6):1014–8.

233. Grubb RL Jr, Raichle ME, Eichling JO, et al. Effects of subarachnoid hemorrhage on cerebral blood volume, blood flow, and oxygen utilization in humans. J Neurosurg 1977;46(4): 446–53.

234. Hino A, Mizukawa N, Tenjin H, et al. Postoperative hemodynamic and metabolic changes in patients with subarachnoid hemorrhage. Stroke 1989; 20(11):1504–10.

235. Voldby B, Enevoldsen EM, Jensen FT. Regional CBF, intraventricular pressure, and cerebral metabolism in patients with ruptured intracranial aneurysms. J Neurosurg 1985;62(1):48–58.

236. Powers WJ, Grubb RL Jr, Baker RP, et al. Regional cerebral blood flow and metabolism in reversible ischemia due to vasospasm. Determination by positron emission tomography. J Neurosurg 1985; 62(4):539–46.

237. Kawamura S, Sayama I, Yasui N, et al. Sequential changes in cerebral blood flow and metabolism in patients with subarachnoid haemorrhage. Acta Neurochir (Wien) 1992;114(1–2):12–5.

238. Yundt KD, Grubb RL Jr, Diringer MN, et al. Autoregulatory vasodilation of parenchymal vessels is impaired during cerebral vasospasm. J Cereb Blood Flow Metab 1998;18(4):419–24.

239. Yundt KD, Grubb RL Jr, Diringer MN, et al. Cerebral hemodynamic and metabolic changes caused by brain retraction after aneurysmal subarachnoid hemorrhage. Neurosurgery 1997; 40(3):442–50.

240. Noske DP, Peerdeman SM, Comans EF, et al. Cerebral microdialysis and positron emission tomography after surgery for aneurysmal subarachnoid hemorrhage in grade I patients. Surg Neurol 2005;64(2):109–15.

Imaging Pathophysiology and Neuroplasticity After Stroke

James M. Mountz, MD, PhD

KEYWORDS

- Imaging • Stroke • Neuroplasticity

There has recently been an increase in imaging technology and imaging methodology enabling noninvasive exploration of brain function to such an intricate degree as to enable measurements of small spatial and short temporal cerebral operations responsible for neurologic and functional recovery after stroke. This development has allowed conceptualization of rehabilitation strategies designed to maximally enhance rehabilitation protocols tailored to the individual patient's deficits. Rehabilitation strategies may now be designed and optimized by using methods to synchronize functional training of brain regions ascribed to those areas innately undergoing neuronal plasticity change responsible for stroke recovery. To apply these noninvasive imaging methods effectively, a clear understanding is needed of the imaging methodologies and how these are best applied to understand brain physiology during the stroke recovery process to provide a solid rationale for development of rehabilitation protocols.

Techniques for assessing perfusion and metabolism include regional cerebral blood flow (rCBF), and 2-fluoro-2-deoxy-D-glucose F 18 ([^{18}F]FDG) positron emission tomography (PET). In addition, hemodynamic vascular insufficiency can be assessed using $^{15}O_2$ extraction PET and rest and Diamox rCBF PET. The status of the periinfarction region can be characterized in components of diaschisis and ischemia using rest/stress rCBF assessment of cerebral vascular reserve.

As the brain recovers from cerebral infarction, areas of reorganization and energy use by the brain can be measured using oxygen extraction methods with PET, [^{18}F]FDG glucose use by PET. Imaging of the stroke recovery process focuses on the physiologic model of stroke characterized by rCBF and cerebral metabolism.

The results of advanced imaging technologies on cerebral damage and cerebral reorganization during rehabilitation can lead to adaptive treatment strategies for rehabilitation. Success can be monitored to assess the optimization of rehabilitation strategy design to maximize neurologic recovery from stroke by using facilitatory methods to maximally synchronize rehabilitation techniques with recovery of functionally counterpart areas of viable brain.

CEREBROVASCULAR DISEASE

Cerebrovascular disease is occurring at a more dramatically increased rate than previously anticipated (730,000 people each year) in the United States.[1] Because of this high incidence and the resulting high percentage of chronic disabilities (approximately 50%–65%), stroke rehabilitation is recognized as a major concern of health care professionals.[2] Despite this recognition, the value and method of rehabilitation in stroke patients remain controversial.[3] Rehabilitation of stroke patients consists of varying combinations of compensatory and facilitatory techniques.

This work was supported by Grant R01 HD32100 from the National Institutes of Health and a Pilot Imaging Program Grant from the Department of Radiology at the University of Pittsburgh.
Division of Nuclear Medicine, Department of Radiology, University of Pittsburgh Medical Center, PET Facility-B-932, 200 Lothrop Street, Pittsburgh, PA 15213-2582, USA
E-mail address: mountzjm@upmc.edu

Compensatory training techniques emphasize attention to unaffected neuromuscular components to improve functional status. Facilitatory techniques attempt to promote or hasten the recovery of affected extremities to a normal movement pattern.

Recently, studies have shown the importance of specific rehabilitation therapies to improve upper extremity function in patients with chronic stroke. The improvement in arm function in patients who underwent specific rehabilitation therapy was attributed to reorganization of cortical networks. Imaging techniques are becoming increasingly important tools for identifying cortical regions underlying functional reorganization, and detection of such areas might become a basis for specific training promoting the optimal reorganization of cortical networks to enhance motor control.[4]

However, because of time constraints and regard to increasing health care costs, rehabilitation of patients with stroke seems to be shifting to a greater percentage use of compensatory techniques in an attempt to obtain a functional level high enough to allow the patient to return to the community earlier. It is unclear how the shift away from emphasis on facilitatory techniques is affecting long-term neurologic and functional recovery. Part of the difficulty studies encounter in attempts to prove the value of stroke rehabilitation in general or the superiority of 1 therapeutic technique to another is because of the heterogeneity of patients with stroke. Another area of difficulty is the lack of understanding of the process(es) of neurophysiologic recovery from a stroke. A major goal of image use in rehabilitation medicine is to identify imaging parameters corresponding to cerebral reorganization to demonstrate an association between neurologic and functional recovery with cerebral reorganizational changes to better understand the stroke recovery process, and allow for better designed rehabilitation strategies that are tailored to the individual patient's deficits.

Imaging techniques can have a significant effect on several areas of implementation of rehabilitation treatment. (1) Prognosis for recovery: by being able to document cerebral reorganization and show an association between neurologic recovery and ongoing cerebral reorganization, it is anticipated that physicians will be able to advise patients and families earlier concerning chances for, and extent of, recovery. Improved ability to provide prognosis will assist patients and families in coping with the disabilities secondary to a stroke and assist in long-term planning for the disposition and needs of the patient. In the present era of increased health care cost containment, accurate prediction of rehabilitation potential will become increasingly important when allocating scarce treatment resources. (2) Imaging techniques can provide a rationale for rehabilitation techniques and criteria for patient selection. Evidence that a functional deficit is rooted in damage, recovery from which seems to require cerebral reorganization, suggests that the use of facilitatory techniques may be the best strategy to optimize stroke recovery.

Selection of imaging techniques directed by rehabilitative outcome provides a rationale for development of physical rehabilitation strategies based on implementation of adaptive plasticity models and allows patient selection into more individualized rehabilitation treatment programs, emphasizing facilitatory versus compensatory techniques. More specifically, a better understanding of the anatomic relationship between neuronal plasticity changes identified by cerebral metabolism and blood flow at rest and areas of cerebral function identified in task activation allows for optimization of rehabilitation strategy design by using methods to synchronize brain regions ascribed to functional training with brain regions undergoing neuronal plasticity change.

PET radionuclide brain imaging methods can also assess neuronal integrity and selective neuronal damage. PET tracers for imaging hypoxia can be used to distinguish tissue in the progress of infarction from tissue that will recover. Functional imaging can also be used to provide information concerning restroke risk and prognosis for recovery from the stroke-induced neurologic deficits in the context of 2 major models of recovery: the resolution of diaschisis and cerebral reorganization in spared brain.

EVALUATION OF CBF, METABOLISM, AND RECEPTORS USING PET TRACERS

The major PET radiopharmaceutical substance used to measure cerebral perfusion is $H_2^{15}O$.[5,6] The major PET radiopharmaceutical substance used to measure regional cerebral metabolism is [^{18}F]FDG.[7] Oxygen metabolism can be directly measured with $^{15}O_2$.[8] Hemodynamic compromise in symptomatic patients with occlusive vascular disease can be identified by cerebrovascular reserve by measuring oxygen extraction fraction (OEF) by $^{15}O_2$ PET, which has been found to be an independent predictor of high stroke risk.[9] Flumazenil C 11 ([^{11}C]FMZ) is a central-type benzodiazepine receptor (BZR) binding agent that has been shown to be a marker of neuronal alterations and selective neuronal loss induced by ischemia.[10,11] The hypoxia agent fluoromisonidazole F 18 ([^{18}F]FMISO) is a 2-nitroimidazole derivative that is selectively trapped in hypoxic viable cells in patients with acute stroke and binds to periinfarct penumbra tissue destined to progress to infarction.[12,13]

METABOLISM, OEF, AND CEREBROVASCULAR REACTIVITY MEASUREMENTS OF PERIINFARCTION TISSUE HEMODYNAMICS

The major PET radiopharmaceutical used to measure regional cerebral metabolism is [18F]FDG.[7,14] The major PET radiopharmaceutical used to measure oxygen metabolism is $^{15}O_2$.[15] Because patient functional outcome depends on CBF, cerebral metabolism, and oxygen extraction after stroke, it is important to understand the current state of knowledge that has been provided by PET to further our understanding of rehabilitation and cerebral reorganization after stroke.

There are several methods for discriminating between an rCBF reduction that represents a primary vascular constraint and that which is a secondary manifestation of reduced neurometabolic activity. One method is oxygen extraction analysis during PET scans, in which it is determined whether a greater than usual percentage of O_2 is being extracted from regions that seem to have reduced rCBF. If the oxygen extraction is abnormally high, then the rCBF reduction represents a vascular constraint to an area with normal metabolism and an ischemic condition exists. If, on the other hand, oxygen extraction is normal, then the rCBF reduction indicates a reduced metabolic rate in the region and is simply reflecting the close coupling between rCBF and regional cerebral metabolism.

Another method is vascular reactivity or stress testing. It has been demonstrated that regions of reduced metabolic activity show an unusual degree of increase in rCBF during CO_2 or Diamox stress.[16–18] The increase is larger relative to that in tissue with normal metabolic rate, probably because of a nonlinearity in vessel response; constricted vessels react more to CO_2 than dilated blood vessels (in the absence of vascular constraints). This finding has been reported previously as the law of initial values[19] and as normalization of the rCBF pattern in Alzheimer disease during CO_2 stress.[20,21] Thus, cerebrovascular reactivity testing typically exaggerates an rCBF defect pattern that is a result of hemodynamic constraints but reduces the pattern abnormality in patients who have rCBF defects arising purely from metabolic or parenchymal reductions in cerebral activity. Because pure diaschisis regions have reduced metabolic activity and blood flow but lack hemodynamic constraint, presence of this reverse

Diamox effect can be used to identify areas of diaschisis and provide a positive prognosis for stroke recovery in such cases.[19]

EVALUATION OF ISCHEMIA BY PET

The major utilities of PET brain imaging in cerebrovascular disease is for diagnosis of critically hemodynamic cerebrovascular compromise that may result in an infarction or chronic ischemia using $H_2^{15}O$ measures of regional cerebral perfusion, $^{15}O_2$ PET measures of decreases in OEF, or ^{11}CO PET measures of increases in regional cerebral blood volume (CBV) associated with compensatory vasodilation in ischemic states.

PET MEASURES OF CBF AND OEF

rCBF is a sensitive indicator of cerebral status outside the infarction region including identification of diaschisis. However, there are some confounds inherent in interpreting normal and reduced resting state rCBF.[22] Decreased resting rCBF may occur as a result of impaired vascular supply (ischemia) or it may reflect reduced neurometabolic activity, such as that resulting from neuronal loss, diaschisis, or other parenchymal dysfunction. It is often difficult to know whether reduced rCBF outside infarcted tissue reflects ischemia, that is, true vascular constraints, or whether it is simply a secondary manifestation of reduced neurometabolic activity caused, for example, by neuronal loss or disconnection effects such as diaschisis. There are several methods for discriminating between an rCBF reduction that represents a primary vascular constraint and that which is a secondary manifestation of reduced neurometabolic activity, as illustrated in **Fig. 1**.[23] Another method is vascular reactivity or stress testing, which can be performed with standard clinical brain single photon emission computed tomography (SPECT) as described earlier, and with PET.

Using PET radiotracers, a sequential, 2-stage classification of chronic hemodynamic impairment for patients with atherosclerotic carotid artery disease, based on experimental data, was proposed.[24,25] As described earlier, stage I (autoregulatory vasodilation) was identified as an increase in CBV or mean vascular transit time in the hemisphere distal to the occlusive lesion with normal CBF and OEF. Stage II (autoregulatory failure) was characterized by reduced CBF and increased OEF with normal oxygen metabolism. These stages were defined originally using PET techniques (**Fig. 2**) in patients with severe atherosclerotic carotid artery stenosis or occlusion and

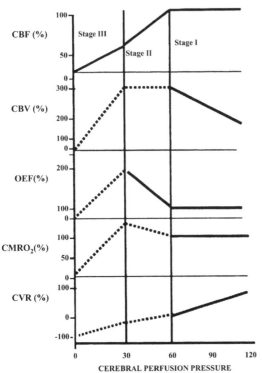

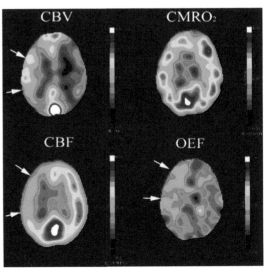

Fig. 2. Stage 2 hemodynamic failure. Increased CBV indicates autoregulatory vasodilation (CBV, *arrows*). This increase is insufficient to maintain flow, however, and flow decreases (CBF, *arrows*). In this situation, the brain can increase the fraction of oxygen extracted from the blood (OEF, *arrows*) to maintain normal oxygen metabolism (CMRO$_2$) and brain function. (*From* Derdeyn CP, Videen TO, Yundt KD, et al. Variability of cerebral blood volume and oxygen extraction: stages of cerebral haemodynamic impairment revisited. Brain 2002;125:596; with permission.)

Fig. 1. CBF, CBV, and OEF in relation to reduced cerebral perfusion pressure (CPP) as might be seen in a slow progressive occlusion of the internal carotid arteries. As the CPP (x-axis) decreases there is an increase in CBV as a result of vascular dilatation, which initially maintains a normal and unchanged CBF and unchanged OEF (stage 1). However, as the limit of vascular dilatation is achieved and the CPP continues to decrease (stage 2), there is a decrease in CBF, which is compensated by an increase in OEF. When the OEF becomes maximal and CPP continues to decrease (stage 3), oxygen and nutrients supplied to the brain cannot be maintained, resulting in irreversible ischemia and infarction. The stages are referenced to the changes in OEF. Stage I, OEF is unchanged. Stage II, OEF begins to increase. Stage III, OEF declines. Solid lines show changes that are known and dashed lines, those that are postulated. (*From* Nemoto E, Yonas MH, Chang Y. Stages and thresholds of hemodynamic failure. Stroke 2003;34(1):2; with permission.)

have been widely applied in the study of human cerebrovascular disease.[26]

TIME-DEPENDENT PROGRESSIVELY EVOLVING STROKE PENUMBRA

In acute ischemic stroke there is a time-dependent progressively evolving penumbra extending from the stroke epicenter through morphologically intact but functionally impaired viable tissue to normal tissue as a result of blood flow reduction

below critical threshholds.[27] During the state of stroke evolution, the tissue at risk of infarction can be identified only by functional imaging. This penumbral tissue can be classified as having a critical flow decrease with preservation of O$_2$ consumption and increased O$_2$ extraction. This misery-perfused tissue has been consistently observed within the first few hours following ischemic stroke but usually develops into necrosis tissue on follow-up observations if treatment is not successful. Pathophysiologic changes that are occurring during the early period after a focal ischemia can be followed by multitracer PET, as this type of imaging provides quantitative maps of important physiologic variables. These changes include rCBF, regional cerebral metabolic rate oxygen, and regional OEF (rOEF), and regional cerebral metabolic rate of glucose, as these changes were studied after occlusion of the middle cerebral artery (MCA) in animal experiments,[28] as shown in **Figs. 3** and **4**.

In a study by Heiss and colleagues[29] PET CBF studies were used within 3 hours of onset to identify the various compartments of the infarct outlined on magnetic resonance (MR) imaging 2 to 3 weeks after a hemispheric stroke in 10 patients. Critical hypoperfusion below the viability threshold accounted for the largest proportion (mean, 70%) of the infarct, whereas penumbral tissue (18%) and initially sufficiently perfused tissue (12%) were responsible for considerably smaller portions of the infarct. This finding indicates that early critical flow disturbance leading to rapid cell damage is the predominant cause of infarction, whereas secondary and delayed pathobiochemical processes in borderline or initially sufficiently perfused regions contribute only little to the final infarct.[30] Emerging therapeutic strategies should be targeted to the initially critically perfused tissue subcompartments. Clinical trials might benefit from stratification of patients for target tissue compartments by applying functional imaging.[29] Functional imaging modalities that could eventually include tracers for neuronal integrity could be used in the future to select thrombolytic therapy. Such techniques may permit the extension of the critical time for inclusion of patients to be managed clinically with aggressive strategies.[27]

PET MEASURES OF CEREBRAL TISSUE VIABILITY STATUS IN ISCHEMIC BRAIN

Recognizing the presence of selective neuronal damage is important when a cerebral revascularization procedure or use of neuroprotective agents for hemodynamic cerebral ischemia is contemplated for therapy. However, it is

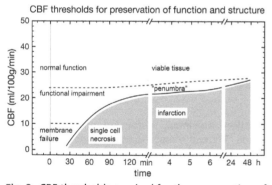

Fig. 3. CBF thresholds required for the preservation of function and morphology of brain tissue. The development of single cell necrosis and infarction depends on the duration of time for which CBF is impaired. The solid line separates structurally damaged from functionally impaired but morphologically intact tissue (the penumbra), and the dashed line distinguishes viable from functionally impaired tissue. (*Reprinted from* Heiss W-D. Systemic rtPA in patients with acute ischemic stroke. 2nd Virtual Congress of Cardiology. Germany, 1998. Copyright © 1999–2001 Argentine Federation of Cardiology. Available at: http://www. fac.org.ar/scvc/llave/stroke/heiss/heissi.htm. Accessed December 8, 2009; with permission.)

important to measure the extent of damaged but viable tissue to weigh benefits versus risks. Imaging of the central-type BZR, which is expressed by most cortical neurons, provides information on the neuronal alterations induced by ischemia in vivo.[31,32]

Central BZR ligands, such as [11C]FMZ, are markers of neuronal integrity and therefore are useful in the differentiation of functionally and morphologically damaged tissue early in ischemic stroke. **Fig. 5** shows a patient example from a [11C]FMZ study showing early identification and treatment of reversible ischemic damage to cortical tissue. In this study, 11 patients with acute hemispheric ischemic stroke were treated with recombinant tissue plasminogen activator and underwent $H_2^{15}O$ blood flow and [11C]FMZ PET within 3 hours of onset of symptoms. Hypoperfusion was always observed but there was substantial reperfusion seen 24 hours after thrombolysis in most patients, as shown in **Fig. 5**.[33]

Hemodynamic ischemia caused by internal carotid artery (ICA) occlusive disease may cause not only borderzone infarction but also selective neuronal damage beyond the regions of infarcts, which may be detected by a decrease in BZR in the normal-appearing cerebral cortex. Yamauchi and colleagues[34] conducted a study to determine whether selective neuronal damage is associated with borderzone infarction in ICA occlusive disease. **Fig. 6** illustrates the results of the study, and shows that in ICA occlusive disease, borderzone infarction is associated with extensive decreases of BZR beyond the regions of infarcts, which suggests that hemodynamic cerebral ischemia may cause selective neuronal damage in the chronic stage. Recognizing selective neuronal damage is important for understanding the pathophysiology of hemodynamic cerebral ischemia in patients with ICA occlusive disease.

Cerebral infarction after ischemic stroke involves a complex series of pathophysiologic changes that evolve in time and space. Hypoperfused, hypoxic, but initially viable tissue is progressively transformed to infarction as a result of a time-dependent cascade of functional and metabolic changes induced by ischemia.[35] The geographic distribution and evolution of tissue hypoxia can be assessed by the PET tracer [18F]FMISO. Markus and colleagues[36] conducted a study of hypoxia in cerebral infarction that found that significantly higher volumes of hypoxic viable tissue were observed in the region corresponding to the center of the infarct in patients studied within 6 hours of stroke onset, whereas in those studied at later times, hypoxic tissue was present mostly in the periphery or external to the infarct.

A

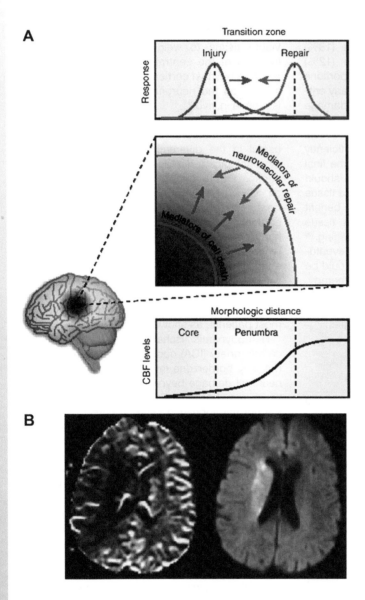

Fig. 4. The stroke penumbra and repair/therapy mechanisms. (*A*) The penumbra is traditionally defined as an area with mild to moderate reductions in CBF (*bottom graph*). Within such areas, spreading waves of death mediators convert at-risk brain tissue into infarction. The new penumbra comprises the transition zone between injury and repair (*top graphics*). Unknowns to be addressed include the levels of blood flow and initial injury corresponding to these transition zones and the regulatory mechanisms and molecular signals in multiple cell types that mediate the switch from injury into repair. These phenomena are highly dynamic. CBF thresholds evolve over time, mediators switch from deleterious to beneficial roles, and injury-repair transition zones may be anatomically heterogeneous with simultaneous mechanisms of tissue decline and recovery. (*B*) The clinically applied imaging penumbra is operationally defined as the mismatch between larger areas of cerebral blood perfusion deficits (*left*) and smaller lesions detected on diffusion-weighted MR imaging (*right*). It will be important to develop and validate new imaging techniques that can help distinguish injury versus repair gradients within these areas of perfusion-diffusion mismatch in stroke subjects. (*From* Lo EH. A new penumbra: transitioning from injury into repair after stroke. Nat Med 2008;14:498; with permission.)

Fig. 7 shows the temporal evolution of hypoxic viable tissue in acute ischemic stroke.

RECOVERY FROM STROKE: DIASCHISIS RESOLUTION AND CEREBRAL REORGANIZATION

In general, 2 competing but not necessarily mutually exclusive models can explain the mechanisms underlying the often-observed recovery of classic neurologic and cognitive function after stroke. One model is that recovery essentially reflects resolution of a temporary cessation of function in brain tissue not directly destroyed by the stroke but nevertheless affected via deafferentation and a consequent diaschisis.[37,38] The second model is that recovery involves spared brain taking on functions previously performed by damaged brain tissue. Thus, the first model emphasizes changes associated with diaschisis resolution, whereas the second entails cerebral reorganization in non-infarcted brain regions.[39]

CEREBRAL DIASCHISIS AS A RESULT OF STROKE

Diaschisis and the role it plays in recovery of function after stroke has a long history starting with Von Monakow's classic article in 1914.[40] Many neurologists can attest that the improvement observed in function after left MCA stroke (eg, progression from hand and leg weakness with aphasia to just hand weakness) seems linked to anatomy adjacent to the cerebral infarction. Von

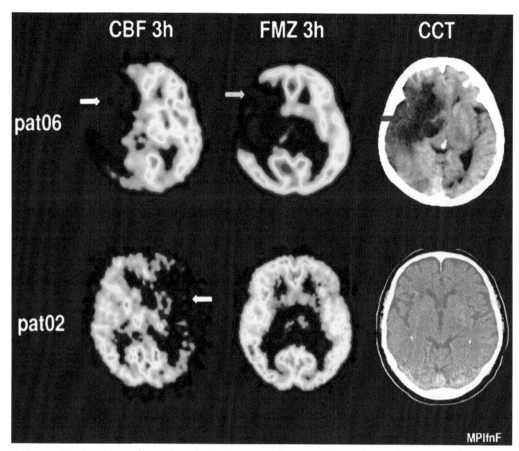

Fig. 5. Two patients who underwent early treatment with recombinant tissue plasminogen (rTPA) activator demonstrate large ischemic areas (*white arrows*). Top row of images shows a patient with a large area of decreased blood flow and corresponding FMZ binding (*blue arrow*) and corresponding large infarction on late cranial CT (*red arrow*). The absence of FMZ binding predicted the absence of tissue viability as confirmed on CT despite infusion of rTPA. Bottom row of images shows a patient with a large area of decreased blood flow but no significant decrease in FMZ binding (*blue arrow*). The presence of FMZ binding predicted the existence of tissue viability that benefited by the infusion of rTPA. The benefit of rTPA in this physiologic state is confirmed by the absence of infarction on late cranial CT. (*From* Heiss W-D, Kracht L, Grond M, et al. Early [^{11}C]flumazenil/ H$_2$O positron emission tomography predicts irreversible ischemic cortical damage in stroke patients receiving acute thrombolytic therapy. Stroke 2000;31(2):368; with permission.)

Monakow defined diaschisis as reduced regional functioning resulting from deafferentation or the interruption of normal input to a region not directly involved in the stroke. PET and SPECT studies have demonstrated remote effects in rCBF consequent to focal infarction.[41] Distinguishing between regional ischemia and depressed neurometabolic activity is aided by calculating rOEF by comparing simultaneous measurements of rCBF and cerebral metabolic rate for oxygen (CMRO$_2$),[42,43] as discussed earlier. Although reports of ischemic penumbra[44] and luxury perfusion[45] persisted post stroke, some studies reported normal oxygen extraction in regions surrounding stroke, suggesting a greater role of diaschisis rather than ischemia in the reduced activity levels.[46] A PET study of 6 stroke patients with motor hemineglect reported significant diaschisis in frontal and parietal cortices ipsilateral to, but outside the infarction. Edema and ischemic penumbra were excluded as likely explanations for most of the observed hypometabolism by measuring normal OEF extraction on ^{15}O$_2$ PET.[47] Cerebral metabolism in the diaschisis region, as measured by local glucose consumption, is also decreased. Using a unilateral carotid and MCA occlusion model in cats, mildly suppressed 2-deoxyglucose C 14 use in the contralateral hemisphere was demonstrated.[48] Thus, diaschisis can involve areas outside the lesion in the affected hemisphere and areas in the other hemisphere (eg, cross-hemispheric or cross-callosal diaschisis).

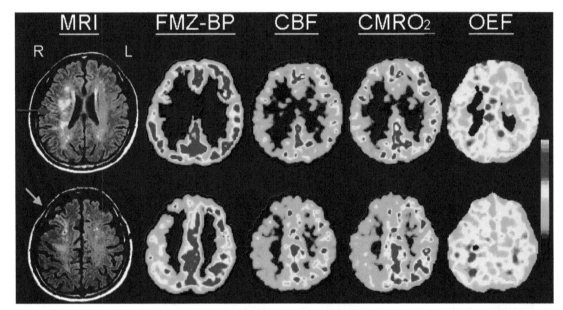

Fig. 6. PET images on 2 different levels show parallel decrease of FMZ binding potential (FMZ-BP), CBF, $CMRO_2$, and an increase of OEF in patient with right ICA occlusion who showed internal borderzone infarction (*red arrow*) with cortical extension (*green arrow*) on corresponding MR images. In addition to markedly reduced FMZ-BP in region with small cortical infarcts, a decrease of FMZ-BP was found in normal-appearing cerebral cortex beyond borderzone infarcts. (*From* Yamauchi H, Kudoh T, Kishibe Y, et al. Selective neuronal damage and borderzone infarction in carotid artery occlusive disease: a 11C-flumazenil PET study. J Nucl Med 2005;46(12):1975; with permission.)

IMPROVEMENT OF STROKE-INDUCED NEUROLOGIC DEFICITS ATTRIBUTABLE TO CEREBRAL DIASCHISIS RESOLUTION

In patients who have had a stroke, the blood flow defect size (Vrcbf) on a blood flow image is typically much larger than the abnormality visualized on computed tomography or MR imaging because the cause of blood flow reduction comprises the sum of diaschisis and chronic ischemia (and possibly other terms) in addition to the stroke defect volume (Vrcbf = $V_I + V_D + V_{MRI}$). A quantitative method to calculate the extent of the rCBF defect size compared with the anatomic stroke volume has been described.[49] The method allows for the calculation of a diaschisis volume (in cubic centimeters) of reduced rCBF on blood flow images that would correspond to an equivalent volume of total loss of blood flow in that location. This defect volume size could then be properly correlated with anatomic tissue volume loss. This method to measure the blood flow defect volume size in unilateral stroke patients involves comparing rCBF in the involved to the uninvolved hemisphere and has been shown to be useful in the determination of a stroke recovery potential as detailed in previous reports.[49,50] A study on

stroke patients supported the notion that patients with a large blood flow defect in the diaschisis region, which improved naturally, or by rehabilitation techniques over time, tended to show an overall better recovery potential from their stroke-induced neurologic deficits.[51]

The application of this method, and the ability to predict a good stroke outcome prognosis, is illustrated in a 76-year-old man who was studied by brain MR imaging and rCBF ([99mTc]hexamethyl-propylene-amine-oxime [HMPAO]) SPECT 4 weeks and approximately 1 year after a left anterior MCA territory infarction (**Fig. 8**). Two initial and 2 follow-up rCBF scans were performed (using the back-to-back low-dose/high-dose protocol). On the 4-week rCBF scan the effective volume of zero perfusion on the resting rCBF scan was calculated to be 68.1 cm^3, whereas the volume on the Diamox challenge scan was calculated to be 14.3 cm^3. The reduction in rCBF volume is expected in diaschisis because of the reverse Diamox effect, which is compared with an MR imaging volume of 13.7 cm^3. The Diamox challenge study indicated that there was no vascular reserve limitation in the stroke penumbra. At 18-month follow-up the effective volume of zero perfusion on the rest rCBF scan was calculated

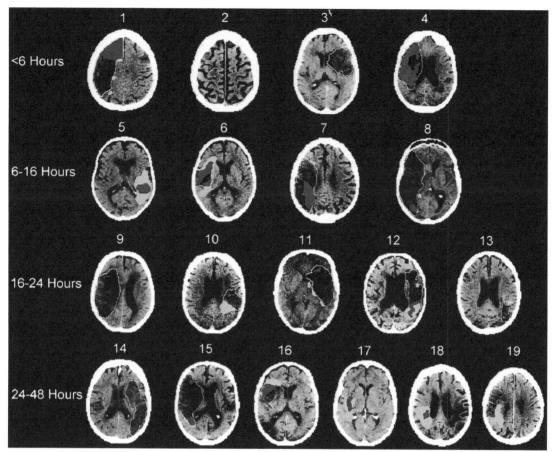

Fig. 7. Representative image slices from several patients showing the region of hypoxic tissue identified by acute-stage [^{18}F]FMISO PET superimposed on the final infarct defined on late CT. Infarct boundary is outlined in yellow. Hypoxic tissue that was viable at the time of acute PET but subsequently infarcted is shown in red; areas that survived are shown in green. Tissue without [^{18}F]FMISO uptake within the final infarct is presumed to have infarcted by the time of the acute PET study. Representative image slice for each patient was chosen to show the maximal extent of hypoxic tissue and therefore does not correspond to center of the final infarct. (*From* Markus R, Reutens DC, Kazui S, et al. Topography and temporal evolution of hypoxic viable tissue identified by ^{18}F-fluoromisonidazole positron emission tomography in humans after ischemic stroke. Stroke 2003;34(11):2649; with permission.)

to be 16.8 cm^3, whereas the volume on the Diamox challenge scan was calculated to be 14.5 cm^3. The significant reduction in rest volume indicates neurometabolic recovery of brain function in the follow-up time period. The patient was administered the Neurobehavioral Cognitive Status Examination, which yields scores in 10 different cognitive domains. The patient experienced substantial cognitive recovery post stroke, as was expected given his substantial area of calculated diaschisis reduction. The patient also had significant recovery in his neurologic status, with near complete recovery in speech and right lower extremity function, and some recovery in his right upper extremity function.

CEREBRAL REORGANIZATION

Cerebral reorganization is a second process to explain recovery of neurologic and cognitive function after stroke. This process involves spared brain areas taking on function previously performed by brain tissue damaged by stroke (eg, the cortical presentation of the hand or other damaged sensory-motor regions) extending into adjacent tissue, or the uninvolved hemisphere takes on the cognitive capabilities of the infarcted side. Experimental evidence for cerebral organization in the sense of uninvolved brain taking on new functions after cerebral infarction is most conspicuously observed in studies of patients recovering from aphasia after sustaining a left hemispheric

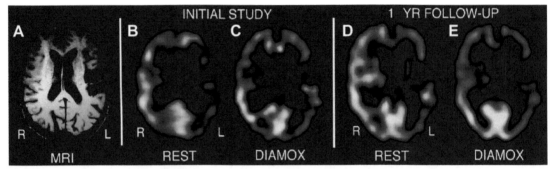

Fig. 8. MR imaging and rCBF SPECT images from a 76-year-old man who was studied by brain MR imaging (*A*) and rCBF SPECT 4 weeks and approximately 1 year after a left anterior MCA territory infarction. Two initial and 2 follow-up rCBF scans were performed (using the back-to-back low-dose/high-dose Diamox vasoreactive stress protocol). The patient underwent follow-up rCBF scanning in an identical manner approximately 1 year post stroke. The 4-week poststroke rCBF scan demonstrates an effective volume of zero perfusion on the resting rCBF scan to be 68.1 cm^3 (*B*), whereas the volume on the Diamox challenge scan was calculated to be 14.3 cm^3 (*C*). This reduction in rCBF defect volume is expected in diaschisis. At 1-year follow-up the effective volume of zero perfusion on the rest rCBF scan was calculated to be 16.8 cm^3 (*D*), whereas the volume on the Diamox challenge scan was calculated to be 14.5 cm^3 (*E*). The recovery of rCBF caused by diaschisis resolution is best seen on the rest image (*D*) at 1 year after stroke compared with the initial rest image (*B*). (*From* Mountz JM, Liu HG, Deutsch G. Neuroimaging in cerebrovascular disorders: measurement of cerebral physiology after stroke and assessment of stroke recovery. Semin Nucl Med 2003;33(1):72; with permission.)

infarction. In 1971 evidence was obtained[52] to suggest the right hemisphere is responsible for improving language function because there was speech arrest in recovering aphasic patients during right carotid injections of amytal. In addition, patients recovering from left hemispheric stroke-induced aphasia who subsequently suffered a right hemispheric stroke once again became aphasic. Early attempts to study this issue with electrophysiologic recordings during language processing and recovering aphasia generated data supporting the view that restoration of language entailed reorganization of brain function with increasing participation of the nondominant hemisphere.[53] More recent imaging studies using PET have produced evidence of increased activity in the contralesional hemisphere after stroke but also indicated there was individual variability in addition to evidence for recruitment of areas outside the infarct and the damaged hemisphere during certain conditions. A single PET study of a recovered aphasic patient showed focal increased activity in a right hemisphere lesion exactly homologous to the left hemisphere lesion during a speech test.[54] In addition, using H$_2$^{15}O PET measures of regional cerebral perfusion it has been shown that there is right hemisphere activation and activation of spared left hemispheric regions during spontaneous speech production in a group of patients recovering from aphasia.[55]

IMPROVEMENT OF STROKE-INDUCED NEUROLOGIC DEFICITS ATTRIBUTABLE TO CEREBRAL REORGANIZATION

Preliminary results from an rCBF study[56] indicate prefrontal perfusion changes are associated with cerebral reorganization and recovery of function after stroke. In this study longitudinal changes in resting state rCBF initially at 6 weeks and again at 6 months were obtained in patients suffering from unilateral MCA territory infarction. Change in rCBF in the contralesional premotor cortex at 6 months compared with 6 weeks after stroke and correlated with change in functional independence measure (FIM) scores. Results showed that the prefrontal contralesional hemisphere involvement in blood flow correlated with improved FIM scores. The increases in resting state rCBF suggest that reorganization associated with recovery of motor skills is associated with neuronal synaptic changes in the prefrontal brain region. The increase in resting state rCBF in the contralesional premotor and prefrontal cortex suggests there is increased synaptic activity during the resting state, postulated to be attributable to long-term neuronal plasticity changes.

Fig. 9 shows a patient example of the findings. The patient shown is a 57-year-old man who suffered a focal subcortical (left posterior internal capsular) infarction. The figure showed an increase in rCBF in the contralesional premotor

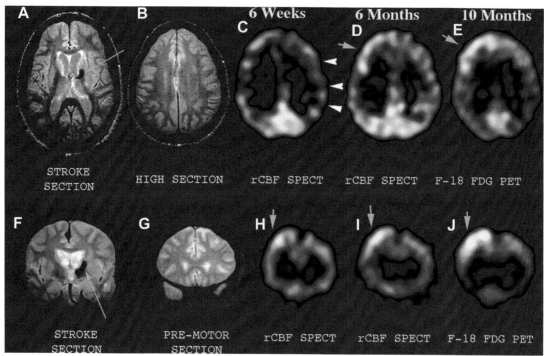

Fig. 9. Increased rCBF and FDG in the contralesional premotor and prefrontal cortex at 6 months after infarction compared with the initial study 6 weeks after infarction. At the 6-month follow-up time the patient dramatically improved from his initial stroke-induced neurologic deficits (6 week FIM = 75/91 to 6-month FIM = 90/91). (*Left*) Images from a 57-year-old man who suffered from a left posterior capsular infarction. (*A*) MR imaging scans in transverse section demonstrating the left posterior capsular infarction (*green arrow*). (*B*) The scout MR imaging used for rCBF SPECT quantification was selected at the level of the centrum semiovale. (*C*) rCBF SPECT scan 6 weeks after stroke. (*D*) rCBF SPECT scan 6 months after stroke. There is increased rCBF in the contralesional premotor and prefrontal cortex (*green arrow*). (*E*) [^{18}F]FDG PET scan at 10 months post stroke. (*F–J*) Corresponding coronal images.

and prefrontal cortex at 6 months after infarction compared with the initial study 6 weeks after infarction. At the 6-month follow-up time the patient dramatically improved from his initial stroke-induced neurologic deficits (6 week FIM = 75/91 to 6-month FIM = 90/91). FDG PET also shows increased metabolism in the contralateral premotor cortex 10 months post stroke.

There is some debate concerning preventing, through intensive motor training, what seems to be additional motor dysfunction that occurs because of longer-term loss of cortical representation areas after the acute stage of stroke.[57] The value and effects of longer-term intervention, even a year or more post stroke, in intense training of affected limbs, is also under debate[58] and may depend on which mechanism of recovery (reorganization or resolution of diaschisis) is operating in individual cases (**Fig. 10**).

ADAPTIVE PLASTICITY IN STROKE RECOVERY

Recent experiments have suggested that bilateral hand motion may facilitate stroke recovery.

Planning and executing bilateral movements after stroke may facilitate cortical neural plasticity by 3 mechanisms: (1) motor cortex disinhibition that allows increased use of the spared pathways of the damaged hemisphere, (2) increased recruitment of the ipsilateral pathways from the contralesional hemisphere to supplement the damaged crossed corticospinal pathways, and (3) upregulation of descending premotor neuron commands onto propriospinal neurons.[59] The extent to which limb exercise can improve function in stroke patients through the mechanism of neural plasticity has major implications for design of individualized rehabilitative training protocols.

One area of difficulty and confound in the investigation of brain changes by functional imaging of cerebral metabolism or blood flow after stroke is the differentiation of patient recovery attributable to (1) underlying resting state changes in brain activity associated with the development of new fields of long-term synaptic activity as separate from (2) brain areas illustrating transient increases in blood flow identified only during task activation, or (3) their interactive effects. This differentiation

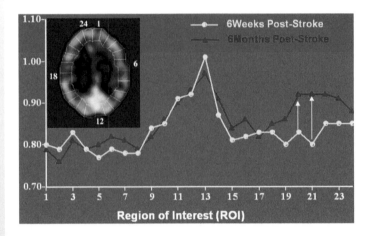

Fig. 10. Circumferential profile plot (24 regions of interest [ROI] of the cortex are generated as shown in small brain diagram) of cortex counts. Plots are average counts per pixel in ROI normalized to whole brain average counts per pixel at 6 weeks (*yellow*) and 6 months (*red*) after cerebral infarction in patient shown in **Fig. 9**. There are increased counts in the contralesional right premotor and prefrontal cortex at 6 months (circumferential profile regions 18–24).

is important when considering the permanency of adaptive plasticity. Based on many neurophysiologic, neuroanatomic, and neuroimaging studies, the cerebral cortex can now be viewed as functionally and structurally dynamic. More specifically, the functional topography of the motor cortex (commonly called the motor homunculus) can be modified by various experimental manipulations, including peripheral or central injury, electrical stimulation, pharmacologic treatment, and behavioral experience. The specific types of behavioral experiences that induce long-term plasticity in motor maps seem to be limited to those that entail the development of new motor skills. Recent evidence demonstrates that functional alterations in motor cortex organization are accompanied by changes in dendritic and synaptic structure, and alterations in the regulation of cortical neurotransmitter systems. These findings have strong clinical relevance as it has recently been shown that after injury to the motor cortex by stroke, postinjury behavioral experiences probably play an adaptive role in modifying the functional organization of the remaining intact cortical tissue.[60]

Prior imaging studies support that contralesional cerebral hemispheric changes are associated with stroke recovery. The proposed underlying mechanisms of cerebral reorganization have been hypothesized to be caused by formation of new neuronal circuitry by neuronal sprouting or synaptogenesis.[61] A more precise understanding of the cerebral areas involved and what neuronal pathways underpinning this cerebral reorganization or the nature of the interplay between ongoing use of the extremity as a result or contributor to this effect has not been comprehensively investigated. It has been recently proposed[62] that to advance our understanding of brain regions involved in the stroke recovery process using neuroimaging measurements of anatomy, baseline CBF and metabolism, and areas of cortical activation are necessary to provide functionally modified maps of (1) the anatomic established areas of motor control (static anatomic scans), (2) semipermanent developing areas of physiologic change (visible on baseline functional scans), and (3) areas of motor activation that may evolve into areas of permanent change (visible on activation scans).

EXPANSION OF CORTICAL REPRESENTATION AREAS AND ROLE OF THE CONTRALESIONAL HEMISPHERE

There is considerable interest in the extent to which cortical representation of hand and other motor functions may remap into adjoining regions following infarction and damage to the primary sensorimotor regions.[63] An experiment in adult squirrel monkeys using intracortical microstimulation measurements showed that after focal ischemic cortical infarctions, skilled retraining of the hand not only prevented the loss of hand representation territory in the adjacent undamaged cortex but also showed that the hand representations expanded into regions formerly occupied by representations of the elbow and shoulder.[57] Additional results from similar studies demonstrated increases in ventral premotor cortex representation after infarction that was in proportion to the amount of hand representation destroyed in the primary motor cortex.[64] These findings suggest that after stroke damage to the motor cortex, rehabilitative training can influence subsequent reorganization in the adjacent intact cortex and supports the notion that undamaged motor cortex may exert an important role in motor recovery.

TASK-DEPENDENT CORTICAL ACTIVATION STUDIES

Blood Oxygen Level Dependent Functional MR Imaging Activation Studies

An understanding of task-dependent cortical activation patterns by noninvasive methods is essential to better understand the several mechanisms presumed to be involved in stroke recovery, such as recovery of penumbral tissues, neural plasticity, resolution of diaschisis, and behavioral compensation strategies.[65] In a study of patients who had right MCA infarctions using near-infrared spectroscopic topography mapping compared with blood oxygen level dependent (BOLD) functional MR (fMR) imaging activation all patients showed right-hand task induced activation of the left sensorimotor and supplementary motor areas as expected but also showed right and left sensorimotor and supplementary motor area activation when performing left-hand motor tasks.[66] Patients with stroke show not only extended activation on the ipsilesional side but also activation of the contralesional motor cortex. In a BOLD fMR imaging study of 11 right-handed left hemispheric stroke patients there was approximately 2.7-fold larger ipsilesional sensorimotor cortex activation ventrally in those with full recovery compared with those with partial recovery.[67] This study illustrates the importance of laterality and the necessity of bilateral hemisphere data acquisition and analysis using regions of interest identified during activation studies in addition to the standard hypothesized regions of motor function.

In a BOLD fMR imaging index finger flexion/extension task paradigm study in patients with stroke the ipsilesional and contralesional cerebral hemispheres showed significant activation of the motor cortex; however, patients with stroke showed that the site of activation was shifted ventrally in the contralesional hemisphere when the unimpaired hand was tested.[68] This finding suggests the presence of contralesional cerebral reorganization as a mechanism of stroke recovery. In a longitudinal study of 8 stroke patients, recovery was accompanied by several patterns of fMR imaging change, with most regions increasing activation over time in the stroke hemisphere. In addition, improvement in clinical outcome was related to increased activation within the sensory cortices of both cerebral hemispheres.[69] Activation of the contralesional cortical motor areas during movements of a paretic hand was shown to represent a functionally relevant, possible adaptive response to brain injury after stroke.[70]

Each fMR imaging task may consist of a block design activation paradigm consisting of 30-second- on and 30-second-off index finger flexion/extension tapping tasks, giving a total scan time of 5 minutes for each task. **Fig. 11** shows a block design task activation paradigm. The activation paradigm was index finger tapping at 2 Hz. These movements were synchronized to a visible tap and test cue displayed by a computer-driven projector to a mirror visualized by the subject. This task was followed by the opposite index finger tapping in the same time sequence. The study consists of 5 pairs of 30-second task and control blocks, separated by 5 minutes of rest with the eyes closed. **Fig. 12** shows the BOLD fMR imaging results for right index finger flexion/extension activation task. **Fig. 13** shows the fMR imaging BOLD results for the right index finger flexion/extension task. All x, y, z coordinates are in the Montreal Neurological Institute (MNI) space.[71]

H₂¹⁵O PET Activation Studies

Normal subject: quantitative dynamic H₂¹⁵O PET hand motion

In the normal subject response to finger tap activation task, the subject underwent sequential rest/tap dynamic $H_2^{15}O$ PET scans with arterial sampling for quantitative blood flow analysis. Data were analyzed using a 1-tissue compartment model to obtain K1 (mL/min/mL) and quantification was expressed in standard units of ml/100 g/min. MR imaging data were coregistered to the $H_2^{15}O$ PET scans by automated image registration (AIR) software (**Fig. 14**).

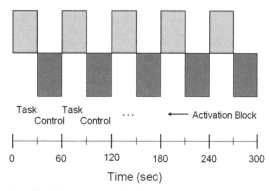

Fig. 11. Block design E-prime task activation paradigm. The activation paradigm was index finger tapping at 2 Hz. These movements were synchronized to a visible tap and rest cue displayed by a computer-driven projector to a mirror visualized by the patient. This task was followed by the opposite index finger tapping in the same time sequence. The study consists of 5 pairs of 30-second task and control blocks, separated by 5 minutes of rest with the eyes closed.

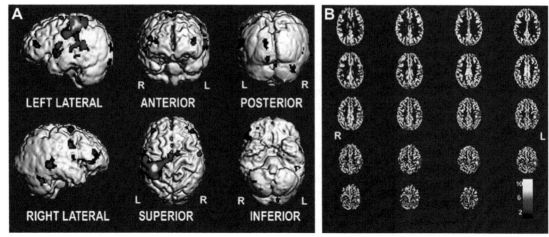

Fig. 12. Right index finger flexion/extension activation task superimposed on (*A*) three-dimensional rendering in patient's PET space (neurologic format) and (*B*) gray matter segmentation images in radiological format. The *t*-value scale of statistical significance for both figures is indicated by the color bar.

Coregistration of BOLD fMR imaging task activation signal region to H$_2$^{15}O PET allows for quantitative of regional cerebral perfusion in regions of significant BOLD fMR imaging signal (**Fig. 15**).

H$_2$^{15}O PET activation studies after stroke

Research in task-dependent cortical activation patterns by noninvasive methods is essential to better understand the several mechanisms presumed to be involved in stroke recovery, such as recovery of penumbral tissues, neural plasticity, resolution of diaschisis, and behavioral compensation strategies.[65] After striatocapsular infarction sparing the cortex, functional brain imaging has consistently documented abnormal patterns of activation during movement of the affected hand, notably enhanced bilateral activation of motor pathways and recruitment of sensory and secondary motor structures not normally involved in the task.[72] In a PET task activation study 5 patients with left striatocapsular infarction were studied twice with PET during right thumb-index tapping tasks, around 2 months (PET1) after stroke and again around 8 months (PET2) after

RIGHT INDEX FINGER TAP

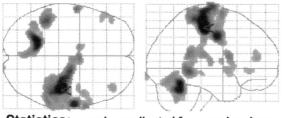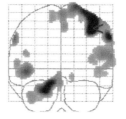

Statistics: *p–values adjusted for search volume*

set–level		cluster–level			voxel–level					x,y,z{mm}
p	c	p corrected	k$_E$	p uncorrected	p FWE-corr	p FDR-corr	T	(Z$_=$)	p uncorrected	
0.000	11	0.000	4126	0.000	0.000	0.000	16.55	Inf	0.000	42 −24 54
					0.000	0.000	11.78	Inf	0.000	62 −8 42
					0.000	0.000	11.69	Inf	0.000	34 −24 72
		0.000	1206	0.000	0.000	0.000	12.92	Inf	0.000	−20 −56 −28

Fig. 13. Right index finger flexion/extension task. For cluster level significance, k$_E$ is the number of contiguous voxels in the cluster with p scores based on the likelihood of finding clusters of this size. For the voxel-wise threshold FWE-corr and FDR-corr are 2 different methods of correcting for multiple comparisons. The T score is the computed T score of the voxel value. For right tapping (x, y, z) = (42, −24, 54) is the left sensorimotor cortex and (−20, −56, −28) is the right cerebellum. These coordinates are in the left finger motor cortex and cerebellum, respectively, in locations typically activated in this task.

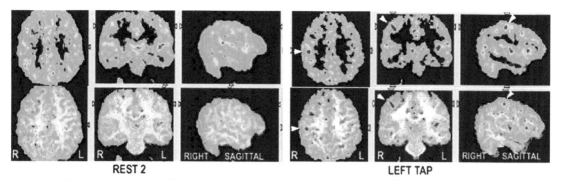

REST 2   LEFT TAP

Fig. 14. $H_2^{15}O$ PET scans. First $H_2^{15}O$ PET scan performed with patient in resting state (*left*), followed by a repeat $H_2^{15}O$ PET scan performed with patient performing left index finger tapping protocol at 2 Hz (*top, right*). $H_2^{15}O$ PET scans were coregistered to MR imaging. Activation is seen in the right motor cortex on $H_2^{15}O$ PET (*white arrow*). On left tap the right motor cortex shows an increased flow from 57.9 mL/100 g/min at rest to 77.8 mL/100 g/min during the task.

stroke.[73] The ipsilesional primary sensorimotor (SM1) activation peak was compared with those from 7 age-matched healthy controls. At PET1 and PET2 there was bilateral motor network activation, as shown in **Fig. 16**.

In a study of patients who had right MCA infarctions using near-infrared spectroscopic topography mapping compared with BOLD fMR imaging activation all patients showed right-hand task induced activation of the left sensorimotor and supplementary motor areas as expected but also showed right and left sensorimotor and supplementary motor area activation when performing left-hand motor tasks.[66] Patients with stroke show not only extended activation on the ipsilesional side but also activation of the contralesional motor cortex. This finding suggests the presence of contralesional cerebral reorganization

as a mechanism of stroke recovery. In a longitudinal study of 8 stroke patients, recovery was accompanied by several patterns of fMR imaging change, with most regions increasing activation over time in the stroke hemisphere. In addition, improvement in clinical outcome was related to increased activation within the sensory cortices of both cerebral hemispheres.[69] Activation of the contralesional cortical motor areas during movements of a paretic hand was shown to represent a functionally relevant, possible adaptive response to brain injury after stroke.[70]

To determine whether fMR imaging signal was correlated with motor performance at different stages of poststroke recovery and to assess the existence of prognostic factors for recovery in early functional MR images, 8 right-handed patients with pure motor deficit secondary to a first

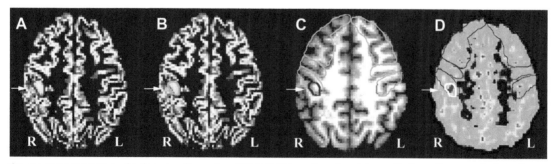

Fig. 15. Coregistration of left index finger tap BOLD fMR imaging signal to spoiled gradient recalled MR image and to the fourth $H_2^{15}O$ (left index finger tap) PET scan. (*A*) BOLD fMR imaging left finger tap activation region (*white arrow*) on segmented gray matter MR imaging scan. (*B*) ROI (*green*) delineated at a *t*-value for statistical significance greater than 2 on BOLD fMR imaging left finger tap activation scan. (*C*) ROI for left- and right-hand motor (M1) left and right premotor (PM), left and right prefrontal (PF) cortexes and the ROI for a *t*-value for statistical significance greater than 2 on the BOLD fMR imaging left finger tap scan. (*D*) BOLD fMR imaging ROI for left index finger task translated to the left index finger tap PET scan. A similar location can be observed for activation in right motor cortex on PET and BOLD fMR imaging left finger tap activation studies.

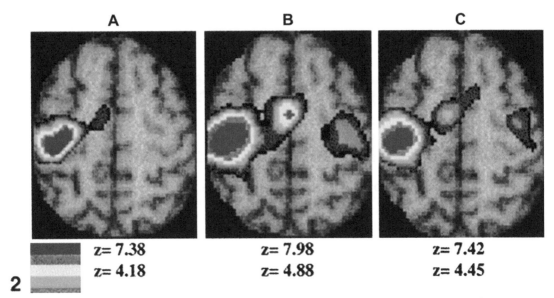

Fig. 16. Group activation patterns during the right thumb-index tapping task at the level of the hand motor cortex, in controls (*A*) and in patients at 2 months after stroke (PET1) and again around 8 months after stroke (PET2) ((*B*) and (*C*), respectively), superimposed on the corresponding MR imaging axial cut from the MNI template. The Z score is also displayed according to the color scale shown. The activation of the contralateral SM1 in patients in both PET studies is larger than controls and extends posteriorly beyond the border of the activation in controls. The figure also illustrates activation only in the contralateral supplementary motor area in controls, whereas in patients there is bilateral motor network activation in both PET studies, more prominent in PET1. (*From* Calautti C, Leroy F, Guincestreb JY, et al. Displacement of primary sensorimotor cortex activation after subcortical stroke: a longitudinal PET study with clinical correla. Neuroimage 2003;19(4):1653; with permission.)

lacunar infarct localized on the pyramidal tract were studied.[74] The intensity of the activation (**Fig. 17**) in the classic motor network (ipsilesional S1M1, ipsilesional ventral premotor cortex, and contralesional cerebellum) 20 days after stroke was correlated with better recovery. The higher the earlier activation in the ipsilesional M1, S1, and insula, the better the recovery 1 year after

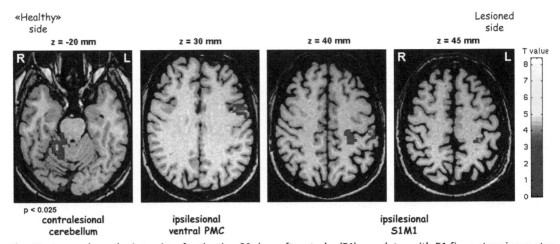

Fig. 17. Areas where the intensity of activation 20 days after stroke (E1) correlates with E1 finger tapping motor performance (statistical parametric mapping regression). Activations are overlaid on a healthy brain. The lesioned side is on the left of the image (radiological convention). The higher the earlier activation in the ipsilesional M1, S1, and insula, the better the recovery 1 year after the stroke. (*From* Loubinoux I, Dechaumont-Palacin S, Castel-Lacanal E, et al. Prognostic value of fMRI in recovery of hand function in subcortical stroke patients. Cereb Cortex 2007;17(12):2984; with permission.)

the stroke. Patients who activated the posterior primary motor cortex early had a better recovery of hand function. This finding suggests that there is benefit in increasing ipsilesional M1 activity shortly after stroke as a rehabilitative approach in mildly impaired patients. These results suggest that patients who are able to activate the ipsilesional primary motor cortex early experience a better recovery and highlight the importance of establishing suitable rehabilitation procedures in the early phase of poststroke recovery.

SUMMARY

Use of imaging with the objective of improvement of stroke recovery should have a significant impact on determination of prognosis for recovery, which should assist patients and families in coping with the disabilities secondary to a stroke and assist in long-term planning for the disposition and needs of the patient. Serial evaluation of stroke physiology and presence or absence of cerebral reorganization by imaging techniques will provide a rationale for development of physical rehabilitation strategies based on implementation of adaptive plasticity models and allow patient selection into more individualized rehabilitation treatment programs emphasizing facilitatory versus compensatory techniques.

ACKNOWLEDGMENTS

The author greatly appreciates the generous support of the staff of the UPMC PET facility and University of Pittsburgh Medical Center MRI research facility. Special thanks to Drs Mathis, Boada, and Price of the Department of Radiology and their staff for assistance with the PET and MR data included in this manuscript, Drs Ricker and Zafonte of the Department of Physical Medicine and Rehabilitative for advice on Stroke Rehabilitation Protocols, and Drs Wechsler, Uchino, and Hammer from the Stroke Center, Department of Neurology for assistance in patient recruitment.

REFERENCES

1. Broderick J, Brott T, Kothari R, et al. The Greater Cincinnati/Northern Kentucky Stroke Study: preliminary first-ever and total incidence rates of stroke amount blacks. Stroke 1998;29:415–21.
2. Anderson TP. Studies up to 1980 on stroke rehabilitation outcomes. Stroke 1990;21:1143–5.
3. Sawner K, LaVigne J, editors. Brunnstrom's movement therapy in hemiplegia: a neurophysiological approach. 2nd edition. Philadelphia: Lippincott; 1992.
4. deBode S, Firestine A, Mathern GW, et al. Residual motor control and cortical representations of function following hemispherectomy: effects of etiology. J Child Neurol 2005;20:64–75.
5. Raichle ME. Measurement of local cerebral blood flow and metabolism in man with positron emission tomography. Fed Proc 1981;40(8):2331–4.
6. Baron JC, Bousser MG, Comar D, et al. Noninvasive tomographic study of cerebral blood flow and oxygen metabolism in vivo. Potentials, limitations, and clinical applications in cerebral ischemic disorders. Eur Neurol 1981;20(3):273–4.
7. Sokoloff L, Reivich M, Kennedy C, et al. The [^{14}C]deoxyglucose method for the measurement of local cerebral glucose utilization: theory, procedure, and normal values in the conscious and anesthetized albino rat. J Neurochem 1977;28:897–916.
8. Raichle ME, Martin WRW, Herscovitch P, et al. Brain blood flow measured with intravenous H$_2$^{15}O. J Nucl Med 1983;24(9):790–8.
9. Nemoto EM, Yonas H, Pindzola RR, et al. PET OEF reactivity for hemodynamic compromise in occlusive vascular disease. J Neuroimaging 2007;17(1):54–60.
10. Dong Y, Fukuyama H, Nabatame H, et al. Assessment of benzodiazepine receptors using iodine-123-labeled iomazenil single-photon emission computed tomography in patients with ischemic cerebrovascular disease: a comparison with PET study. Stroke 1997;28:1776–82.
11. Sasaki M, Ichiya Y, Kuwabara Y, et al. Benzodiazepine receptors in chronic cerebrovascular disease: comparison with blood flow and metabolism. J Nucl Med 1997;38:1693–8.
12. Read SJ, Hirano T, Abbott DF, et al. Identifying hypoxic tissue after acute ischemic stroke using PET and 18F-fluoromisonidazole. Neurology 1998;51:1617–21.
13. Read SJ, Hirano T, Abbott DF, et al. The fate of hypoxic tissue on 18F-fluoromisonidazole positron emission tomography after ischemic stroke. Ann Neurol 2000;48:228–35.
14. Huang SC, Phelps ME, Hoffman EJ, et al. Noninvasive determination of local cerebral metabolic rate of glucose in man. Am J Physiol 1980;238:E69–82.
15. Mintun MA, Raichle ME, Martin WR, et al. Brain oxygen utilization measured with O-15 radiotracers and positron emission tomography. J Nucl Med 1984;25:177–87.
16. Mountz JM, Deutsch G, Khan SH. An atlas of regional cerebral blood flow changes in stroke imaged by Tc-99m HMPAO SPECT with corresponding anatomic image comparison. Clin Nucl Med 1993;18:1067–82.
17. Mountz JM, Deutsch G, Kuzniecky R, et al. Nuclear medicine annual. In: Freeman LM, editor. Brain

SPECT: 1994 update. New York: Raven Press; 1994. p. 1–54.

18. Deutsch G, Mountz JM, Liu HG, et al. Cerebrovascular stress tests in parenchymal versus vascular disease. J Nucl Med 1996;37:37–88.

19. Rogers RL, Meyer JS, Mortel KF, et al. Age-related reductions in cerebral vasomotor reactivity and the law of initial value: a 4-year prospective longitudinal study. J Cereb Blood Flow Metab 1985;5:79–85.

20. Bonte FJ, Devous MD, Reisch JS, et al. The effect of acetazolamide on regional cerebral blood flow in patients with Alzheimer's disease or stroke as measured by SPECT. Invest Radiol 1989;24:99–103.

21. Deutsch G, Halsey JH Jr, Harrell LE. Regional CO_2 reactivity of cortical blood flow in Alzheimer's disease. J Cereb Blood Flow Metab 1991;11:S22.

22. Yudd AP, Van Heertum RL, Masdeu JC. Interventions and functional brain imaging. Semin Nucl Med 1991;21:153–8.

23. Nemoto EM, Yonas H, Chang Y. Stages and thresholds of hemodynamic failure. Stroke 2003;34(1):2–6.

24. Powers WJ, Press GA, Grubb RL Jr, et al. The effect of hemodynamically significant carotid artery disease on the hemodynamic status of the cerebral circulation. Ann Intern Med 1987;106:27–34.

25. Derdeyn CP, Videen TO, Yundt KD, et al. Variability of cerebral blood volume and oxygen extraction: stages of cerebral haemodynamic impairment revisited. Brain 2002;125(3):595–607.

26. Baron JC, Bousser MG, Rey A, et al. Reversal of focal "misery-perfusion syndrome" by extra-intracranial arterial bypass in hemodynamic cerebral ischemia. A case study with 150 positron emission tomography. Stroke 1981;12(4):454–9.

27. Heiss W-D, Graf R, Grond M, et al. Measurements of acute stroke events and outcome: present practice and future hope. Cerebrovasc Dis 1998;8(Suppl 2):23.

28. Heiss W-D. Systemic rtPA in patients with acute ischemic stroke. 2nd Virtual Congress of Cardiology. Germany, 1998. Available at: http://www.fac.org.ar/scvc/llave/stroke/heiss/heissi.htm. Accessed December 8, 2009.

29. Heiss W-D, Thiel A, Grond M, et al. Which targets are relevant for therapy of acute ischemic stroke? Stroke 1999;30:1486–9.

30. Lo EH. A new penumbra: transitioning from injury into repair after stroke. Nat Med 2008;14:497–500.

31. Sette G, Baron JC, Young AR, et al. In vivo mapping of brain benzodiazepine receptor changes by positron emission tomography after focal ischemia in the anesthetized baboon. Stroke 1993;24(12):2046–57.

32. Nakagawara J, Sperling B, Lassen NA. Incomplete brain infarction of reperfused cortex may be quantified with iomazenil. Stroke 1997;28:1124–32.

33. Heiss W-D, Kracht L, Grond M, et al. Early [^{11}C]flumazenil/H_2O positron emission tomography predicts irreversible ischemic cortical damage in stroke patients receiving acute thrombolytic therapy. Stroke 2000;31(2):366–9.

34. Yamauchi H, Kudoh T, Kishibe Y, et al. Selective neuronal damage and borderzone infarction in carotid artery occlusive disease: a 11C-flumazenil PET study. J Nucl Med 2005;46(12):1973–9.

35. Dirnagl U, Iadecola C, Moskowitz MA. Pathobiology of ischemic stroke: an integrated view. Trends Neurosci 1999;22(9):391–7.

36. Markus R, Reutens DC, Kazui S, et al. Topography and temporal evolution of hypoxic viable tissue identified by ^{18}F-fluoromisonidazole positron emission tomography in humans after ischemic stroke. Stroke 2003;34(11):2646–52.

37. Seitz RJ, Azari NP, Knorr U, et al. The role of diaschisis in stroke recovery. Stroke 1999;30:1844–50.

38. Calautti C, Baron JC. Functional neuroimaging studies of motor recovery after stroke in adults: a review. Stroke 2003;34(6):1553–66.

39. Mountz JM, Liu HG, Deutsch G. Neuroimaging in cerebrovascular disorders: measurement of cerebral physiology after stroke and assessment of stroke recovery. Semin Nucl Med 2003;33(1):56–76.

40. Von Monakow C. Diaschisis, brain and behavior. In: Pribram KH, editor. Mood, states and mind. Baltimore, MD: Penguin; 1969. p. 27–36.

41. Feeney DM, Baron JC. Diaschisis. Stroke 1986; 17(5):817–30.

42. Herold SB, Broen MM, Frackowiak RS, et al. Assessment of cerebral haemodynamic reserve: correlation between PET parameters and CO_2 reactivity measured by the intravenous 133 xenon injection technique. J Neurol Neurosurg Psychiatr 1988; 51(8):1045–50.

43. Ackerman RH, Alpert NM, Correia JA, et al. Positron imaging in ischemic stroke disease. Ann Neurol 1984;15(Suppl):S126–30.

44. Astrup J, Siesjo BK, Symon L. Thresholds in cerebral ischemia: the ischemia penumbra. Stroke 1981;12: 723–5.

45. Baron JC. Positron tomography in cerebral ischemia: a review. Neuroradiology 1985;27:509–16.

46. Raynaud C, Rancurel G, Samson Y, et al. Pathophysiologic study of chronic infarcts: the importance of the peri-infarct area. Stroke 1987;18:21–9.

47. Fiorelli M, Blin J, Bakchine S, et al. PET studies of cortical diaschisis in patients with motor hemineglect. J Neurol Sci 1991;104:135–42.

48. Ginsberg MD, Reivich M, Giandomenico A, et al. Local glucose utilization in acute focal cerebral ischemia: local dysmetabolism and diaschisis. Neurology 1977;27:1042–8.

49. Mountz JM. A method of analysis of SPECT blood flow image data for comparison with computed tomography. Clin Nucl Med 1989;14(3):192–6.

50. Dierckx RA, Dobbeleir A, Pickut BA, et al. Technetium-99m HMPAO SPET in acute supratentorial ischaemic

infarction, expressing deficits as millilitre of zero perfusion. Eur J Nucl Med 1995;22(5):427–33.

51. Mountz JM, Modell JG, Foster NL, et al. Prognostication of recovery following stroke using the comparison of CT and Tc-99m HM-PAO SPECT. J Nucl Med 1990;31(1):61–6.

52. Kinsbourne M. The minor hemisphere as a source of aphasic speech. Arch Neurol 1971;25:302–6.

53. Papanicolaou AC, Moore B, Deutsch G, et al. Evidence for right hemisphere involvement in recovery from aphasia. Arch Neurol 1988;45(9):1025–9.

54. Buckner RL, Corbetta M, Schatz J, et al. Preserved speech abilities and compensation following prefrontal damage. Proc Natl Acad Sci U S A 1996;93:1249–53.

55. Ohyama M, Senda M, Kitamura S, et al. Role of the nondominant hemisphere and undamaged area during word repetition in post-stroke aphasics. Stroke 1996;27:897–903.

56. Chu WJ, San Pedro EC, Hetherington HP, et al. Post-stroke cerebral reorganization in human brain identified by 31 P MR spectroscopic imaging and F-18 FDG PET. J Magn Reson Imaging 2002;15(5):1243–8.

57. Nudo RJ, Wise BM, SiFuentes F, et al. Neural substrates for the effects of rehabilitative training on motor recovery after ischemic infarct. Science 1996;272:1791–4.

58. Taub E. Increasing behavioral plasticity following central nervous system damage in monkeys and man: A method with potential application to human developmental motor disability. In: Julesz B, Kovacs I, editors. Maturational windows and adult cortical plasticity. Redwood City (CA): Addison-Wesley; 1995. p. 201–15.

59. Cauraugh JH, Summers JJ. Neural plasticity and bilateral movements: a rehabilitation approach for chronic stroke. Prog Neurobiol 2005;75:309–20.

60. Nudo RJ, Plautz EJ, Frost SB. Role of adaptive plasticity in recovery of function after damage to motor cortex. Muscle Nerve 2001;24:1000–19.

61. Dijkhuizen RM, Ren JM, Mandeville B, et al. Functional magnetic resonance imaging of reorganization in rat brain after stroke. Proc Natl Acad Sci U S A 2001;98:12766–71.

62. Thirumala P, Hier DB, Patel P. Motor recovery after stroke: lessons from functional brain imaging. Neurol Res 2002;24:453–8.

63. Seitz RJ, Freund HJ. Plasticity of the human motor cortex. Adv Neurol 1997;73:321–33.

64. Frost SB, Barbay S, Friel KM, et al. Reorganization of remote cortical regions after ischemic brain injury: a potential substrate for stroke recovery. J Neurophysiol 2003;89:3205–14.

65. Kwakkel G, Kollen B, Lindeman E. Understanding the pattern of functional recovery after stroke: facts and theories. Restor Neurol Neurosci 2004; 22:281–99.

66. Kato H, Izumiyama M, Koizumi H, et al. Near-infrared spectroscopic topography as a tool to monitor motor reorganization after hemiparetic stroke: a comparison with functional MRI. Stroke 2002;33(8):2032–6.

67. Zemke AC, Heagerty PJ, Lee BA, et al. Motor cortex organization after stroke is related to side of stroke and level of recovery. Stroke 2003;34:e23–8.

68. Cramer SC, Finklestein SP, Schaechter JD, et al. Activation of distinct motor cortex regions during ipsilateral and contralateral finger movements. J Neurophysiol 1999;81:383–7.

69. Nhan H, Barquist K, Bell K, et al. Brain function early after stroke in relation to subsequent recovery. J Cereb Blood Flow Metab 2004;24:756–63.

70. Johansen-Berg H, Dawed H, Guy C, et al. Correlation between motor improvements and altered fMRI activity during rehabilitative therapy. Brain 2002; 125:2731–42.

71. Evans AC, Collins DL, Mills SR, et al. 3D statistical neuroanatomical models from 305 MRI volumes. Proc IEEE Nucl Sci Symp Med Imaging Conf 1993:1813–7.

72. Calautti C, Leroy F, Guincestre JY, et al. Dynamics of motor network overactivation after striatocapsular stroke: a longitudinal PET study using a fixed-performance paradigm. Stroke 2001;32:2534–42.

73. Calautti C, Leroy F, Guincestreb JY, et al. Displacement of primary sensorimotor cortex activation after subcortical stroke: a longitudinal PET study with clinical correlation. Neuroimage 2003; 19(4):1650–64.

74. Loubinoux I, Dechaumont-Palacin S, Castel-Lacanal E, et al. Prognostic value of fMRI in recovery of hand function in subcortical stroke patients. Cereb Cortex 2007;17(12):2980–7.

Index

Note: Page numbers of article titles are in **bold face** type.

A

Adaptive plasticity, in stroke recovery, 117–118

Aging, normal brain imaging in, 4–10

Alzheimer's disease
  amyloid ligands for, **33–53**
  dopaminergic ligands for, 68
  dopaminergic neuron imaging for, 75–82
  early diagnosis of, **15–31,** 16–17
    amyloid ligands for, 20, 22
    comparative studies of, 22–23
    differential diagnosis, 25–26
    FDDNP ligands for, 22–23
    FDG studies in, 16–18, 23
    limitations of, 24–26
    Pittsburgh compound-B ligands for, 20–23,
      35–36, 38–41
  novel ligands for, 72
  populations at risk for, 17, 19–20

Amino acid transport, aging effects on, 10

[^{11}C]-Aminocyclohexanecarboxylate, for brain
  imaging, aging effects on, 10

Amyloid, deposition of, in Alzheimer's disease,
  33–35, 40–42

Amyloid ligands, for dementia, **33–53**
  Alzheimer's, 20, 22, **33–53**
  apolipoprotein E and, 40
  carbon-labeled, 36–37
  fluorine-labeled, 37–38
  need for, 41–43

Antibodies, monoclonal, to amyloid, for dementia, 35

Aphasia, recovery from, 116

Apolipoprotein E, in Alzheimer's disease, 17,
  19–20, 40

Arterial occlusive disease, 86–89

Atherosclerosis, carotid artery, 92

Atrophy, brain, age-related, 8

[^{18}F]-AV45 (Florpiramine), for Alzheimer's disease, 37

[^{18}F]-AV-133 (^{18}F]9-fluoropropyl
  dihydrotetrabenazine), for dopaminergic neurons,
  76–80

[^{11}C]-AZD2138, for Alzheimer's disease, 37

[^{18}F]-AZD4694, for Alzheimer's disease, 38

B

[^{18}F]-BAY94-9172 (Florbetaben), for Alzheimer's
  disease, 37

Benzodiazepine receptors, aging effects on, 9

Beta cells, pancreatic, ligands for, 79–80

[^{11}C]-BF227 benzoxazole derivative, for Alzheimer's
  disease, 36–37

Blood flow, cerebral. *See* Cerebral blood flow.

Blood volume, cerebral
  control of, 86
  in carotid artery occlusion, 87–89

Brain imaging
  after stroke, **107–125**
  amyloid ligands for, **33–53**
  for atypical parkinsonism, **65–74**
  for cerebrovascular disease, **83–125**
  for dementia, **15–31, 33–53**
  for Parkinson disease, **55–64**
  normal patterns and variants in, **1–13**
    artifacts and, 4
    auditory activation, 3
    eyes open or shut, 3
    higher cognitive processes, 3–4
    in infants, 4–5
    in normal aging, 8–10
    technical factors, 4–9
  vesicular monoamine transporter type 2 targeted
    in, 66, **75–82**

^{125}I-Bromostylrylbenzene, for dementia, 35

C

[^{11}C]-Carbon monoxide, for post-stroke changes,
  108

Carotid artery
  atherosclerosis of, 92
  occlusive disease of, 86–89

Carotid Occlusion Surgery Study, 83, 87

Cerebellar hypometabolism, in infarction, 92–93

Cerebral blood flow
  after stroke, 108–110, 114–117
  aging effects on, 5–6
  control of, 84–86
  in carotid artery occlusion, 87–89
  in infarction, 89–93
  in intracerebral hemorrhage, 94
  in subarachnoid hemorrhage, 94–97
  in vascular dementia, 94
  normal, 83–84

Cerebral blood volume
  control of, 86
  in carotid artery occlusion, 87–89

Cerebral metabolic rate of glucose, normal, 84

Cerebral metabolic rate of oxygen
  after stroke, 108–109
  in carotid artery occlusion, 87–89
  in infarction, 89–93

PET Clin 5 (2010) 127–130
doi:10.1016/S1556-8598(10)00036-2

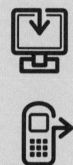

Printed and bound by CPI Group (UK) Ltd, Croydon, CR0 4YY

03/10/2024

01040351-0016